The Essential Guide to

Self Harm

ROBERT DUFFY SERIES EDITOR

Published in Great Britain in 2019 by

need2know

Remus House
Coltsfoot Drive
Peterborough
PE2 9BF
Telephone 01733 898103
www.need2knowbooks.co.uk

Contents

Introduction **5**

Self Harm Vs. Suicide 6
Warning Signs 6
Symptoms of Self Harm 8

Not Only Suicidal Thoughts 9
Summary 11

Chapter 1: Definitions **13**

Self Harm in the Past 13
Professional Issues 15

Despair 18
Summing Up 21

Chapter 2: Bullying **23**

Being Bullied 23
Telling 26
Doing Something About It 27

Re-Inventing 28
Summing Up 30

Chapter 3: Your Reflection **31**

The Media 31
The Social Group 32

Summing Up 35

Chapter 4: Peer Pressure **37**

Risk Taking 38
I Need to Be Liked 40

Summing Up 43

Chapter 5: Difficult Children **45**

Education 45
With Others 47

The Family 47
Summing Up 49

Chapter 6: Mental Health Issues **51**

Early Adulthood and Adolescence 51
A Cry for Help 53
Talking to Someone – Counselling 53

Support 55
Professional Support 57
Summing Up 60

Chapter 7: Families 61

Being Tough but Fair 61
Parents 62
Significant Others................................. 63
The Kids 64

Friends 65
Seeking Support 66
Summing Up 67

Chapter 8: The Professional Point of View 69

Listen Up 70
Facilitating a Group............................. 71

Summing Up 75

Chapter 9: Loving Yourself 77

Needs and Wants 78

Summing Up 85

Chapter 10: Good Health and Its Promotion 87

How Do We Stay Healthy? 87
More about Exercise 89
How Can I Improve My Mental Wellbeing? 90

Moving On.. 91
Summing Up 93

Chapter 11: Discussing Our Activities 95

Activity One 96
Activity Two.. 96
Activity Three....................................... 97
Activity Four... 98
Activity Five 99
Activity Six 99

Activity Seven 100
Activity Eight.. 100
Activity Nine... 102
Activity Ten 103
Activity Eleven..................................... 104

Help List 106

Emergency Helplines 106

Glossary 110

Sources 112

Introduction

Adolescents and young people, especially males, are the groups most likely to struggle with self-harm. But these are not the only people who can be affected. There are certain factors, and these will be dealt with in their turn, but we will also give some attention in this book to the questions that families ask, when they find that a young family member has begun to self-harm.

It may initially seem like a clear-cut issue but, the reasons for **self-harm** occurring are far from simple. In this book, we look at the likelihood of surviving this unhappy time in family life – for all concerned. We answer questions family members might have and discuss the different ways forward providing sources for support.

As you read this book, before moving on, each chapter will give you an exercise or scenario which you are asked to read and consider. Your answers will be a reflection of your own knowledge and experience. The final chapter of the book will return to these exercises and explore them in detail. There are no right and wrong answers, so don't worry if your answers differ from those given in the book. That is no bad thing, and the more we can keep an open mind, in dealing with self-harm, the better.

You may also find that your answers change as you read through the book, as many of the questions are based on preconceptions and opinions.

If you want to expand your knowledge, this book includes lots of references for further reading which are perfect for parents, health professionals and students. It would be all too easy to read weighty **psychiatric** tomes, which only emphasise doom and gloom. The recommended reading has been chosen based on the merit that it does not lose sight of the positive outcomes, and offers clear guidance and support.

There are some words here which have slipped into common usage, but which may have a different meaning in a medical context. The glossary at the back of the book will provide explanations of any words that appear in **bold** type. Often these words won't mean exactly what you think they do, so it's best not to assume that you don't need to use the glossary.

Self Harm Vs. Suicide

A suicide attempt is different from self harm, and 'cutting' has many other facets. It is important to distinguish the underlying thinking, so that the help that is offered is appropriate to needs. Suicidal thoughts and suicide are often believed to be the driving force behind self-harm, but it's important to recognise that they aren't necessarily always related. We are all different.

Suicidal thoughts may however be present, or may develop.

Progression to suicidal thoughts is quite a big leap, and in some cases self-harm may provide a sort of safety valve which allows the individual to feel pain and to suffer, but to go no further than that. If they are not suicidal, it would be very wrong to suggest the label to them, as it may become a self-fulfilling prophecy. To think this is to miss the point.

Support and assistance can be offered, however, if suicidal thoughts do become an issue. The emotional vulnerability of anyone who is self-harming is undoubtable, and they are bound to have some unhealthy thoughts about themselves. The degree of pain perceived is a very subjective thing, though, so in medicine it is important to follow the old adage that 'pain is what the patient says it is'.

Thinking that someone should be able to cope with their problems is easy when you're looking at their life from the outside, but nobody can truly judge someone else's emotional pain. Therefore, when we listen to someone who feels like self harming, we give them space to express their fears and feelings, and ask them to say what they think is going on.

The only perception of the pain that really matters is that of the sufferer. There are no magic wands, but the starting point must always be in sight. It is down to the sufferer to explore what has led them to where they are and what is happening. This starting point needs to be in place before any other issues can be resolved.

Warning Signs

Thinking about – or even carrying out – self harm is a fairly likely outcome for anyone who is truly struggling to cope with daily life. It can be a slow, lengthy process or a very short step indeed. Each of us will have a different threshold for what moves us from thinking about self harm to trying it.

Risk taking is a warning sign, and is also a type of self-harm. Anyone who describes themselves as 'useless' or their life as 'pointless' is also very much at risk. (Please note – shouting at them or demanding change is unlikely to help.) Warning bells should start to ring if someone begins to describe themselves as "trapped". This says that they feel trapped into living in a way that is not actually their choice.

This is a sign that their mind is already moving over to negative thinking.

Certain types of **obsessive-compulsive (OCD)** behaviour may be classified as self harm. Finally, there is a surprising amount of peer group pressure involved in some kinds of self harm, and adolescents in particular may find themselves part of a sub-culture where they prove that they are 'hard' – or just one of the gang – by cutting themselves. Can it be assumed that this type of self harm does not express mental anguish? This will be addressed in a later chapter.

Rationalising the things a person does as their "duty" is a less recognised warning sign for self harm. The sense of 'duty' may extend to work as well as family commitments. These include trying to please someone who is never going to be happy, whatever you do. This is not exclusive to older people. In some ways this can be seen as an **addiction**, but it is worth remembering that for intelligent adolescents, their education is their work, and they may be feeling that there are extreme pressures upon them to succeed.

In the long term, feeling that you have no real control over your actions can be really damaging, as the way to good **mental health** is to feel some sense of power and control over the events of life. Feeling anxious or ashamed about a lack of achievement is not unknown for someone who loves their work (to the exclusion of other things in life), and these people can easily become obsessed with their careers and start feeling bad if they spend any time at all away from work.

Trying to cope with impossible relationships can also lead to this feeling of being trapped, as can family commitments which trap us, and eventually destroy any sense of self-worth and value we have. This is a route many of us will go down if we're trying to care for a sick partner or family member. The truth is, being a long-term carer means that life must revolve around the needs of another person.

Time that should be spent exploring and growing into their own strengths and personality, for a surprising number of adolescents, is instead spent acting as carers within the family.

No specific cause has so far been identified for **generalised anxiety**, sometimes described as "free-floating". It can be that we are simply not ready to admit to the cause, even to ourselves. That isn't to say it's not possible to identify a cause in some cases, however. It can just be incredibly difficult – examining the problem.

Someone who has always been sporty and adventurous may move subtly into the practice of putting themselves at risk, before others really begin to notice. Failing to pay proper attention to safety procedures, when engaging in dangerous activities like extreme sports, can be a warning sign. In times of war, if someone becomes depressed, the opportunities to put oneself at risk are massive.

Another way to self-harm is by using drugs or drinking dangerous amounts of alcohol. Substance abuse is a highly dangerous practice, since aerosol sniffing can kill or cause permanent brain damage very quickly. Sniffing damages brain cells, even if it does not kill. There is no doubt that some of us cross a line into excessive use – even if the activities were recreational to begin with – once life takes a turn for the worse.

There's no way to know for sure if today will be the day it all goes down the drain. Always remember that once brain cells are damaged or lost through substance abuse, they cannot be regained or regenerated.

While OCD is extremely distressing, and interferes with life massively, it only really becomes self-harming when the compulsion involves features such as scrubbing with potentially toxic substances, or self damage such as systematic hair pulling. This is certainly self harm, and the main issue is the compulsion to act. A lengthy course of psychotherapy is often required to treat OCD, which is a very difficult **syndrome** to live with.

Behavioural work which aims to re-learn patterns of behaviour is necessary, as well as working to figure out the causes of the disorder. Some people with OCD will be prone to pulling their own hair out strand by strand, which is a harmful behaviour which needs to be resolved. The way back to health for those with the condition is to deal with each compulsion completely.

Other approaches are necessary in cases involving peer pressure, where the cause is different and therefore the solution should be too.

Why is someone going down that route? We'll discuss all of these warning signs in much more detail in later chapters. But what is important is to recognise that these are warning signs, and respond to them by making space for self-expression. The characteristics of some warning signs may well overlap. It's important to address the whys and wherefores of each one once the individual has been able to express the way they are feeling.

Symptoms of Self Harm

The impulse to self-harm is usually kept a secret from friends and family, at least for a while. We do not want to accept the reality of the situation. Eventually the activities become visible, but this may take quite some time, and a considerable amount of serious damage may have been done.

There are differences in the favourite ways of self harming, between men and women. There are many different ways to harm oneself other than cutting – though it's generally the first symptom we'll think of. Other symptoms that count as self-harm include self-burning, and damaging the body by punching, banging, or throwing it against something hard.

Males are more physical, and have more of a tendency to excessive risk taking. **Eating disorders** are more common in women, as is intentionally taking too many tablets. At times, however, people of all genders will use all different approaches to self harm. This is simply a generalisation. Some people will prefer to self harm by sticking things into the body or swallowing objects (such as forks, razors, etc.).

The things that they do tend to make many sufferers feel ashamed or guilty.

Not Only Suicidal Thoughts

The body can be damaged or life threatened by other things within the context of self harm – such as eating disorders and risk-taking – and it is important to examine these. In some ways these are more subtle approaches to self-harm, and they do follow a different path from cutting.

No matter how much evidence there is to the contrary, for example, someone with **BDD (Body Dysmorphic Disorder)** will believe them to be repulsive, disfigured and unlovable. It can be treated successfully, but because incorrect perceptions are in place, it can be hard for the sufferer to understand that they need help to change their thinking. They will begin to feel that life is "pointless" as a result of this distressing syndrome, and may starve themselves to increasingly dangerous levels or become suicidal because they believe there is no hope for them.

Later on in the book, we'll discuss some of the approaches families and partners will need to take in these situations, such as "tough love".

That anxiety, depression and suicide are linked to self-harm is a known fact. Good mental health requires that we all have some time and space for ourselves, and that our lives are not completely subsumed into that of another. Life can become seriously imbalanced if someone is a long-term carer for someone else, even if they are deeply loved. Of course they need help, guidance and support.

Unfortunately, if a carer becomes depressed enough to begin considering self harm, he or she may then feel that it is important that their dependent is not left to the mercies of others, after they are gone. This is a scenario that can often involve a great deal of guilt. The result can sometimes be a murder-suicide or murder-suicide attempt, in which the carer kills the person they care fore before also killing themselves.

So what's going on in these situations? We need to figure out answers to this question.

A 'cry for help' is always important, and should never be ignored. Anxiety can have a crippling effect on everyday life. Some sources claim that only 15-20% of people who self harm could be categorised as mentally ill. Their feelings are often a normal response to what has become an intolerable situation.

In further chapters, we'll discuss the links between self harm and mental illness in greater detail. It's important to keep in mind that depression can come in various forms and severities. What we do know is that a higher proportion than 15-20% of those who self harm go on to attempt suicide, a fact that supports sources that put the amount of self-harmers with depression higher than this percentage.

In this book, we'll use terms like "sufferers" to refer to individuals, rather than "patients". This is because many people who self harm can't really be categorised as patients. Of course, the 15-20% can be referred to as 'patients', but it is impossible to tell, at first glance, who might fall into this category. Discussing the key issues in their life and talking honestly and freely will be a vital aspect of the healing process for these people.

When faced with a young person who has deliberately damaged themselves, many parents will begin to panic and it's easy to understand why. This only leads to increasing the distress and isolation of the self-harming person. Family relationships do not need to become strained, though. Later in the book, we'll look at ways forward so that responses can be calm and sensible.

Labels can be self-fulfilling, and can cause long and lasting damage to someone's life. It is often unnecessary to pin a psychiatric label on individuals who engage in self harm. Proceeding carefully is the best course of action.

Activity

1   Give some thought to the reasons you decided to read this book. Write down any specific questions that you would like to be discussed. As you work through the chapters you may find information that surprises or even challenges you. Be sure to leave a space under each so that you can fill in the answers as you come to them.

2   Write down any reasons you can think of that a person might start self harming.

3   Take note of anything you come across that surprises you or challenges your preconceptions.

Summary

- When you read this book, you'll quickly find that your experience is far from uncommon. While it focuses mainly on support and guidance for the families who care for individuals who self harm, this book also has some useful information for the individuals themselves.

- Health professionals will benefit from the insights that are offered here – which have been drawn from actual people.

- There is a lot of life after self harm.

- Many practices develop into self-harming when life becomes difficult, and perhaps changes direction.

- There is a better, healthier way to live life, and each of the following chapters will help all concerned to find a way forward.

- We should always be careful to avoid having a negative influence on those around us.

- We all have the power to change someone's life for the better.

- We have a massive effect upon those around us – perhaps much more than we realise.

- A key issue in many cases of self harm is the individual's lack of a sense of control over their life.

- A happier and more fulfilling life is possible with proper help and support, and understanding of the situation. You will find a way to move forward.

- To protect the privacy of those who kindly allowed us to share their stories, we have changed the names in all case studies in this book.

- If you self harm, know that your life will not always be like this and you will have a better life that you can look forward to.

Disclaimer

The results of self harming are far ranging, and cause considerable further serious issues, within health care. (Trevillon K et al, 2011).

This book will allow us all to feel more confident about addressing the issues, professional or lay person alike. If we make an effort, we have the potential to help someone who self harms back to a fuller, healthier and happier life, however uncomfortable we may feel addressing the problem initially.

Please note that this book should not be used as a replacement for professional help and counselling. It is meant only as a general guide.

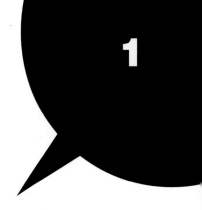

1

Definitions

Self Harm in the Past

The history of self-harm is hidden in the social and world events of particular times, each of which bring their own stressors to everyday life. There are frictions in human society, and sometimes – for great lengths of time – we may find ourselves struggling to find a comfortable place in the world. In Hogarth's images of 'Gin Lane' we saw people who were so overcome by poverty and despair that their only recourse was to drink themselves into the grave.

Whenever individuals speak about the urge to self-harm, they often suggest they 'wanted the pain to prove that they could feel something'. They feel that their responses are not as they should be. Words have failed them, or it has not been possible to find someone to talk to, safely. Living in a social group can sometimes bring with it certain stresses, so as long as civilised human beings have recorded history, individuals have been prone to the possibility of depression.

In the **pathologies** of previous times, how individuals have responded to these stresses may have been a little different to how we respond today, but it is possible to see variations in almost all of the possibilities listed in Chapter One over the centuries. Perhaps this is because the potential for coming to this point is there within all of us.

Symptoms of **paralysis** were sometimes produced in Victorian times when middle class young ladies took to their beds with the 'vapours' and started eating dangerously little. If these young women were alive in the twenty-first century, their retreat from the world into a career of ill health would no doubt be seen as evidence of depression, and there's little doubt that they would be experiencing similar – if slightly different – symptoms no matter what century they lived in.

Throughout history, there have been cases of people no longer caring about survival in times of war and conflict, and acting without regard for self and survival.

Whatever its appearance, self harm has always been around – it's just hidden in a variety of disguises.

Affect is a medical term for emotional response. A "flattening of **affect**" is a term used by doctors to describe the loss of feeling many of those who engage in self harm are experiencing. When individuals begin to feel cut off from the world and from everyday feelings about it, affect is said to have been flattened because their emotions are not registering normally. These changes in emotional response leave the sufferer feeling that they are separate from the world and its events, and then to beliefs that they are different, usually in a negative way.

PTSD, depression and stress all have a tendency to produce this "flattening of affect". This may be the result of bullying, extreme pressure at work or school, family expectations, and so on. The constant feeling of worthlessness brought on by these conditions can cause some sufferers – but not all – to begin to hallucinate, particularly hearing voices which tell them to self harm. Not always, of course.

Auditory hallucinations, in which someone hears voices, are very distressing. The only way to quieten the voices is to comply.

Some features of self harm in history are more subtle than others in appearance, while others can be seen again and again within certain peer groups.

Whatever its appearance, self harm has always been around – it's just hidden in a variety of disguises.

Professional Issues

These feelings and reactions can get in the way of acting as we should, when someone needs us to be there for them. (Grant, Biley, Walker, 2011)

Horror, throughout history, has always been the initial reaction of human beings on discovering a self harm attempt. You may well feel angry, hurt, betrayed and completely confused. As professionals, we may feel guilty and believe that we have failed in what we try to do. The potential waste of life is appalling to us because we feel that life should never come to this deliberate self damage.

When they were most in need of help, many sufferers have reported being treated in a very unsympathetic manner. After all, medical professionals are human beings too, with their own hidden fears and anxieties. This doesn't excuse an unprofessional response to a crisis situation, but it does go some way toward explaining it. An assumption that someone is 'attention seeking' and therefore might be dismissed as not really in trouble is an easy answer, but in fact completely inappropriate.

Nurses who work in Learning Disability may find that someone in their care begins to self-harm. When someone appears in the emergency rooms, having self-harmed, he will be met by nurses trained in the adult branch who have not necessarily had the guidance and training needed to deal with self harm. Uncertainties may translate into apparent callousness.

A medical professional's compassion can sometimes become overwhelmed by fear, as many people fear the idea of self harm. A compassionate response is necessary for all cries for help, however, so it's important that the professional is able to come to terms with their own fears and prevent them from affecting their treatment of patients.

Handling situations involving self harm can also be confusing and challenging for paramedics, who also report that they have no specific training in this.

For any health professional, the adage that we should 'walk a mile in their shoes' is often repeated, but very hard to do. We are also asked to reflect on our practice. What has brought the patient to this point is all too readily discounted in some emergency rooms and mental health wings, where nurses are overworked and all too aware of the "revolving door".

These patients are sometimes treated in a less thoughtful manner than is expected, as the nurses become frustrated with them.

Listening is not something that certain types of nurses see as their remit, and those that do may be conscious that there are others who need their attention. Nurses are asked to always remember that the people they deal with are in need of help, and individual nurses are asked to learn empathy during training. A lack of time very quickly becomes the go-to excuse for nurses, who begin to cite the fact that they are too busy to practice empathy.

Every health professional should examine their own instinctive responses to self-harm, honestly. What you find there may surprise you. We all have our failings, and it's important to recognise that this applies to professionals, too. Whatever your natural response to self harm, it's a good idea to examine the reasons for that response.

Activity

Think about the following questions.

- What sort of feeling is produced when you are faced with evidence of self harm?
- When dealing with situations involving self harm, what are the words that you habitually use?
- How do you act or physically respond to these situations?
- Does your facial and body language suggest a sense of scorn or superiority?
- Do you always use positive and acceptable phrases?
- Is this more marked in certain situations or with certain (types of) individuals?

Whenever someone comes to a point in their career when they believe themselves to be perfect (or even very good!) in their practice, they should recognise that a time to stop and reflect is very, very necessary. It should always be recognised that we can all improve as professionals.

The Group as a Potential Cause of Self Harm

A need to express pain is often present when someone self harms, and usually the person is suffering in some way.

This is not always the case, however. In some peer groups, self harm becomes something fashionable to do, and identifying with these peer groups can result in 'cutting' becoming the norm. How much it hurts has been a matter for discussion in many places. At many other levels, self-harm is kept secret. To want to belong to something so badly that you are prepared to damage yourself is something of an extreme reaction to life.

It becomes a way of proving that you are 'hard', and the group may regard this as a badge of honour.

It's important not to assume that those who self harm for this reason aren't also experiencing some form of mental or emotional pain. It hurts to cut yourself, so it's not something people will do for no reason.

When we talked to 'Harriet', she explained that in much the same way that people of her aged experimented with soft drugs, alcohol, smoking and sex, they also experimented with cutting. These were all things that (it was felt) everybody should try once. She knew that 'most' of her friends were cutting themselves, and became aware that there was 'a sort of competition' going on. She admits that she herself made a conscious effort to build up her tolerance to pain when she tried cutting herself, and tells us that (like her friends) she began to do this in a very small way at first.

We will return to the power of peer group pressure in Chapter Four.

People outside of a group like this may not be aware that this is even happening. Although groups of young people may feel like this is something that binds them together into a kind of identity, they won't share it any further.

It may seem amazing that pain or self harm can become addictive, but what appears to be certain is that those who find they need to damage themselves more and more have a tendency to addictions in the first place. The physiology that underpins self harm reinforces this. The tendency to the development of a type of addiction is sometimes illustrated by this type of self harm.

A person prone to self harm and other addictions may be any combination of insecure, emotional, stressed, intelligent or obsessive. The problems that life throws at us when any of these descriptions apply can easily put us at risk of becoming addicted to something as a way of overcompensating for this reduced control. Addictions are hard to break, even when they take us beyond a point where life is at risk.

People often say that they feel 'more alive' when they put themselves at risk, by whatever means. At this point, self-harm is not a social issue, but has become a symptom of despair. A sense of pleasure can actually be released in the brain when our skin is cut, as our bodies release **endorphins** as part of the healing process. When we do something particularly risky or scary, endorphins are also released alongside adrenaline. This type of high is however just as addictive as any other chemical rush. Again, this is due to the release of endorphins.

For some, the goal is to create a sensation that 'outweighs the internal emotional pain', and some describe a sense in which the pain of the cut (or other damage) makes them feel as though they are at least 'able to feel something'. Feelings that are very difficult to deal with and even more difficult to express have built up inside, and cannot readily be expressed.

Despair

A sense of despair is often what is being expressed when solitary (and often lonely) individuals begin to self harm. If they are faced with realities that are not acceptable to them, they can suffer a great deal of internal conflict, and perhaps also denial and possibly **projection**. The unacceptable truth may be about sexuality, the condition of the family or the loss of ideas, ideals or a belief system. The collapse of a relationship, which was central to the individual's world, may be one example.

As adolescents and young adults figure out where their place might be in the wider world, self harm can often become an issue, as these people are still discovering who they are.

No matter how compelling the evidence, if someone is in **denial** they will refuse to admit – even to themselves – that anything is wrong. Adolescents are not the only group who experience this, of course. Learning that what was once certain in life is no longer the case as situations change in later adulthood can produce similar feelings.

'Jackie' described the build-up of her emotions as 'feeling as if she was going to explode'. On one dark day, she found herself experimenting by turning a knife upon her own arm, and found that this drastic act 'took her somewhere else'. This gave her a 'sense of relief' – a common statement among those who self-harm. She had been concerned that someone might get in her way just as her emotions ran out of control, and that she might accidentally harm them. The tension that she felt seemed to be relieved in some strange way, though, by the pain.

The terrible feelings she had now were less than the originals. She began to feel that she was at least partly in control now, because the pain she was feeling was self-inflicted. The shame and guilt she felt about her desire to cut herself felt somehow more manageable than her original feelings of guilt and shame about the situation she was in. Jackie was 'punishing herself before someone else did', and that made her feel as though she was in control of the situation.

The thought that punishment is a certainty, which arises from guilt and confusion, is a very common one. It is important to recognise that there may be no real need to feel guilty about anything. We will return to this point later, when we look at treatment, because work that is done on returning thinking to a more realistic place is always a good first step.

This is also true if an individual fears the loss of a key relationship – a fear that may well be groundless. Self-harming individuals are sometimes heard to say 'Well, at least there's one thing I can succeed at…' Individuals become desperate, because they do not know where to turn for help.

It becomes difficult to know what to trust, as the world constantly changes and moves away from whatever provided an anchor or comfort for the individual as a child. Figuring out who to turn to for guidance or support can become impossible. In individuals who feel the need to regain some control over the world or their life, self harm can become a handy crutch.

Inflicting pain or damage on oneself is one way of 'showing them'. (Grant et al, 2011) The world now presents terrific uncertainties for these individuals, and although self harm may seem strange to those who haven't experienced it, it is in fact a severe way to get back on top of all of this.

When faced with deeply unacceptable feelings, "Bill" explains that there was a sense in which he was 'detached from the world and from his body' as a means of emotional denial. Like many others, he managed to avoid the pain of the memory, but the result was that he felt emotionally numb. A long period of abuse was the underlying trauma in this case. Convincing himself that it had never happened became Bill's new goal. He wanted to feel alive again, and cutting himself seemed to be the only way to do this.

The thought that punishment is a certainty, which arises from guilt and confusion, is a very common one. It is important to recognise that there may be no real need to feel guilty about anything.

Feeling that you've taken charge of your own justice and the possibility of suffering can often provide people with a sense of control, which can make difficult situations seem easier to deal with.

Dangerous ideas like this often begin as perfectly normal, fixed mental attitudes which are allowed to grow out of proportion.

Activity: Practising Empathy

If you believe that others are denigrating your feelings, or even laughing at them, you will find that the situation is much more difficult to cope with.

- Picture a very difficult time you've gone through, when several bad things may have happened very close together. The events themselves may not have been the worst possible things in your life, just consider your feelings. Perhaps the difficulty came from people around you failing to respond or act in a sympathetic manner. You will find that your emotional pain increases if you have a sense of being trapped in a bad situation and cannot see who to trust or turn to.

- Next, think about how you would like people to have responded to you, and what you would have liked to have happened. What would you like them to say to you? What would make you feel less alone at this time? What should the people be saying?

- How would you like to be treated in a situation like this?

Summing Up

- At some time in our lives, we'll all experience the depths of despair. We may end up feeling permanently afraid if this lasts for a long time, and we'll start feeling trapped. We may consider attempting to harm ourselves if it seems like that's the only option. But there is always another way forward.

- There is always a way out of despair, and it's important that the sufferer remembers this and considers the possibility of help. Being able to believe that help is possible forms a vital first step to recovery, as one of the key aspects of despair is the overwhelming sense of futility.

- Showing consideration to someone who is self harming can allow them to gain some sense of a significant 'other' who cares about them, even if it isn't a perfectly successful interaction. The individual's self-esteem can begin to benefit if they can manage to get the 'right' response from someone else, and this will allow them to – at one level – begin to take control of the situation.

- If we can identify some of the actions, feelings and responses that would make us feel better about life, it is possible to approach someone else, with those responses in mind. If we know how we would like them to respond, we can ask the questions that will give us the right response.

- The exercise in this chapter asks readers to empathise with that dark condition. However, it can also be used by someone who is already on the slippery sole. If an individual can manage to pause, and imagine how he or she would like to be responded to, and what would be good if it happened, two things can be achieved.

2

Bullying

Being Bullied

While bullying is a very sad fact of modern life, it is also possible to recognise that it can be dealt with – either as the target, or as someone who is slipping into the habit of bullying. Probably everyone in the world has at some time been the target of a bully. When it comes to self harm statistics, bullying is a hugely important factor. Even those who habitually bully others are likely to have been bullied in the past.

Activity

- Remember a time when you have been the target of a bully. They may have been in your family, at school or in the workplace. To start this exercise, take note of your role in the situation, where it took place and how old you were.

- Consider the person in the role of "bully".

- Who were they to you? What was their role?

- In what way were they bullying you?

- How did the situation pan out?

- Do you feel any anxiety or sadness about the memory?

- If that person was in front of you now, what would you say to them?

- Now that life has moved on, how would you describe your bully's character?

- Did you recognise what they did as bullying at the time?

For now it is important to examine how unpleasant the experience of being bullied can be. Later in the book, we'll explore the possibility that you may also have made someone's life uncomfortable. At the time, you may not have thought of it as bullying, but as "acting in their best interests" or "building their character". Among children, this may take the form of petty activities such as stealing or pinching or endless nasty remarks.

Everyday life within a family is also controlled by one person who likes to be in charge. What is more surprising is that they get away with it. Every day of the week, you're likely to be able to spot at least one child acting like this.

Acceptance of unpleasant behaviour means that it continues, and always becomes worse. Parents are almost always oblivious, and many never reprimand the child who is behaving badly. The idea that this is simply what the other child does is often something the child who is targeted – even if they are older and bigger – has become resigned to. Some children (and their parents) might even be proud of this type of bullying behaviour.

The bullying child increases his unacceptable behaviour, and grows into an adult who bullies others. (Clarke, 1999) (Dellasega, 2005) Writing from her own experience, Molly Clarke points out that children need clear boundaries and are in fact looking for them. Clarke describes how her personal decision to change her own approach surprised her class, and led to improved classroom activity, as well as greatly improved attitudes from the children.

Acceptance of unpleasant behaviour means that it continues, and always becomes worse. Parents are almost always oblivious, and many never reprimand the child who is behaving badly.

A bully's need for control will eventually lead him to be left alone and lonely. The children in these situations have boundless potential, but no boundaries are ever set which would allow them to reach it. Or they may be uncertain and the source of confusion. Genuine affection and closeness, whatever else happens for a child who was allowed to bully, are often missed out on altogether.

They will never have the chance to become a fully rounded adult who enjoys successful relationships, because the habit of bullying becomes entrenched. In the exercise we were asked to recall what it is like to be bullied. There are two factors that make bullying important in the context of self harm. That a bully can drive their victim to self harm or worse – the first factor – is no real surprise, as this person's life is being made miserable.

The power that bullies wield is always out of proportion to what they do. It is easy for anyone outside the scenario to dismiss what is happening as being of no consequence, but if we do this, we collude with the bully, and cut off another avenue where people can reach out and trust.

But with no habits in place that will help them to cope with being thwarted, the bully becomes the second factor when they learn that their strategies will not always work. Bullies can end up turning upon themselves physically when their anger and frustration with the world become internalised and intensified.

The victims of bullying can be left with severe psychological damage. And the damage that is done is compounded by the failure of those around the situation to act.

However slight the bullying may be, we should always make a stand against it, wherever we see it.

According to the Department for Education, some groups are significantly more likely to be bullied. These include:

- younger children (those aged 10 to 12 years);
- those with a long-term illness or disability;
- those living in the most deprived areas;
- those who had truanted from school in the previous 12 months;
- those living in one-adult households. (DfE, 2018)

However, bullying is not confined to our early years.

Telling

The first step in dealing with a bully is to recognise that something can be done. Those who are being bullied need to confide in someone with authority, and as we tend to think of bullying as an adolescent or childhood event, we think of 'telling your parents'. This looks daunting to begin with, and a person whose self-esteem has been damaged will not initially want to become 'confrontational'.

In the workplace a person targeted by a bully is made to feel like a child, uncertain of their ground, insecure, and unable to achieve. All too often, bullying is handled poorly by those in authority, and this is the case wherever it takes place. This is a short-sighted attitude, however, since an un-checked bully will develop and expand his activities, causing more and more problems as time goes by.

In surveys conducted in working environments, it was found that as many as one in three professionals state that workplace bullying has happened to them. In this case the victim finds himself set impossible targets, which cannot be achieved, and may be publicly mocked for failing. Even in the NHS, 20% of staff report to have been bullied by other staff to some degree, and 43% report having witnessed bullying in the last 6 months. (Carter et al, 2013)

People in positions of authority should be available for these people to turn to. But in some cases, the bully can be the manager themselves. The bully becomes more encouraged and entertained by the distress that is caused. Self-esteem goes through the floor, as a result of the cruel games that the bully plays. It's common to feel that you have no one to turn to if you're being bullied, and most targets quickly come to feel that they have no right to complain. If this becomes the case it should be no surprise that life can become so miserable that we begin to self-harm.

A grievance procedure is in place in the majority of firms, however. A union rep can advise, or there may be someone in the human resources department who can help. There should be someone in your company who is able to remain impartial while providing important advice as someone who understands the procedure.

1-in-5 of all young people has witnessed bullying within the past 12 months, with 50% of them witnessing at least once a month. (Ditch the Label, 2018) Children need boundaries, and they need adults to set them (Clark 1999). It is not unknown for teachers to see the situation as someone else's problem if the target is a child, even if the school is actively approached about the issue.

The situation develops into one in which the teachers feel intimidated by a child or group of children. However, even more serious problems for the school may occur if the bully is allowed to proceed, as they are not only damaging the mental health and progress of their peers but also putting themselves at risk of moving on to more serious activities. It is very difficult to recover from this sort of situation.

When we abdicate our responsibilities in boundary setting, we have abdicated our role as manager, parent or teacher. If someone in an office is destroying team morale and achievement, the manager needs to recognise that they, too, are being manipulated by someone who simply enjoys making others unhappy.

Doing Something About It

To fix a young person with a stare and simply say 'Don't do that' is certainly to invite verbal abuse. If the child or young person being abusive is accompanied by their parent, very often that person will say nothing at all, and will choose to pretend that nothing has happened.

But the fear that underpins this thought – of physical violence – is extremely unlikely. Opportunities are often missed to correct an unpleasant situation, unfortunately, because human beings tend to shy away from actions they view as confrontational. And sometimes these situations are confrontational. But that discomfort is often as bad as it will get – when anyone challenges their behaviour, young people who have never learnt that there are boundaries in life are often too amazed to do anything about it.

Most children have no idea what to do, if people do not crumble before their demands. Errant behaviour will often evaporate if we can steel ourselves to meet abuse without panic and with a quiet smile.

Always remember that in many situations nothing needs to be said if a child is behaving badly in public. They're very likely to turn away and crumple in embarrassment if they're responded to with quiet disgust by a total stranger.

It's also important to refuse to accept verbal abuse from an adult, and the best course of action is to report it to the manager or other authority if it takes place in a public location (such as a shop). Support usually follows. It could potentially be against the law for the manager not to be supportive, and they are likely to be aware of this and insist that the person leaves.

The thought of standing up to a bully, and staying calm, gives a tremendous sense of achievement. The person who has to face down a bully will often be quite surprised if they are able to act in this way under pressure.

When dealing with a bully, then, making sure that someone else knows what has happened is the very first step. The second step is to let them know that their behaviour is not acceptable. Finally, we should figure out if there is anything we can do to decrease repetitions by looking at ourselves. The third step is to start thinking of yourself as someone who is not afraid. This is not easy to do, but very possible.

Re-Inventing

Some people appear to send a message that they can provide fun for bullies – it is sometimes said that we might attract bullying, either through something we say or do. The more cowed and unhappy someone becomes, the more that a bully will attack them. The misery of others is something that bullies thrive on.

When dealing with a bully, we're often advised to re-invent ourselves. The beginning of re-invention lies in the first two steps, outlined above.

Bullies are not immune to put-downs. Scorn is also effective, especially the quiet variety. Perhaps this is rooted in the bully's own insecurity – an already present fear that they do not even admit to themselves. If you had the chance, it might be possible to plan out in advance the things you would like to say to a bully. They may like to get their digs in first, but that doesn't mean you just have to accept the things they say.

Many bullies will not continue if they receive an assertive and confident response to their attacks. They may always hate you, but at least it will be because you stood up to them, rather than because they have you marked as a victim.

A change arising in another (especially the target) is enough to make them unsure of their ground. What has changed? Bullies are often caused to pause when faced with the apparent disappearance of fear from the victim's face and demeanour. They need to feel in control of any situation, so the uncertainty that this change creates is very worrying to them.

The bully will begin to run out of possibilities at this point. Some will attempt to redouble their efforts, but will give up if they are still met with a blank calm rather than distress.

The changes that can happen can have another level for someone who self harms because life has become unbearable in this way.

'Yasmin' began to self harm because of her experience of being bullied by a 'team' of three other girls. As well as a pain that could compete with the pain caused by the others, the damage and pain she caused herself was (in her mind) a way of hurting herself 'before they did' and that it was also a sort of punishment for being unable to cope.

When she decided she'd had enough, Yasmin began only addressing herself to the person she had identified as the leader of the three. She began to role play someone who did not care. Although she was nervous to the point of shaking, she managed to carry off her new image long enough to sow doubt in the leader's mind. The other two not even worthy of her notice, she had decided.

She took to slipping into the part she wanted to play, the part she had practiced again and again in private, whenever the bullies made their appearance. The leader found herself unusually alone, and faltered in her attack. Once the leader had been dissuaded, there was no trouble shaking off the other two – natural followers. The attacks stopped completely soon after, though it wasn't an instant cure for the situation.

In effect, she had re-invented herself, and changed from someone who believed herself to be a victim, into a person with a degree of self-respect. It took Yasmin a long time to realise she 'did not need to (self harm) any more', having acquired the habit when the bullying was at its worst.

The need to cause herself damage and discomfort disappeared once she had learned to respect herself. She was not particularly artistic, but decided to take up sewing and embroidery. Soon, Yasmin was regarded in a very different light by her classmates, having taken to putting her energy into sports and hobbies rather than self harm.

Summing Up

- The despair that causes individuals to harm themselves is all too often caused by bullying.

- This category includes anyone whose actions or lifestyle put them at risk.

- It is important to change the view that we carry of ourselves, but also to accept that sometimes the only real solution is to change our environment completely by leaving it behind.

- If we can practice this, when we move on to new places and situations, we do not carry with us the attitudes and body language that might invite or attract a new set of bullies.

- It is possible to break the dreadful cycle that life becomes, when we are the victims of a bully.

- While cutting remains the most likely response to bullying, there are many other ways to hurt one's self.

3

Your Reflection

The Media

Body ideals are promoted to the extent that some individuals believe they must be thin at all costs, even to the point of risking life. If someone seriously dislikes their body, it is a short step to punishing it. There is no doubt that the media holds a great deal of responsibility for the ways in which we see our bodies, an issue that is forever tied to the concept of self harm.

Self-harm may be fuelled by anger as well as despair, and when anger takes over, it may seem to be the only way to reassert control in life. Although it's no less damaging than cutting or risking an excess of pills, alcohol or any substance, eating disorders are a more subtle form of self harm and develop over a length of time. It quickly becomes irrelevant that the disorder is causing pain or sickness.

Those who starve themselves into illness and disability are making a decision to change themselves, in the belief that this will be an improvement. The logic of the process is powerful and hard to escape, even though it is actually faulty. No truly conscious choice is made in the development of an eating disorder, and it's important that we don't make the mistake of thinking this.

Treating the body badly when we don't like what we see in the mirror can sometimes seem like the only way forward. But it is faulty thinking, which insists that drastic measures are called for. This individual may put themselves at risk in other ways, using chemicals, alcohol or dangerous activities.

Control is often the main goal when it comes to eating disorders. Starving can essentially become addictive once this process has established itself as a habit, as the body's chemistry has changed so radically.

Family, friends and classmates may be seen as not respecting the individual, and this lack of respectability can become all they see when they look in the mirror. Young men may risk their lives on motorbikes at this point, but risk-taking behaviour is by no means limited to males. Proving that they are 'hard' or 'strong' becomes overwhelmingly important.

While it is facile to say that upbringing and background are bases for risk taking, there is no doubt that some who damage themselves as a result of excessive risk are subliminally trying to prove something to a significant (and perhaps absent) figure from their lives. In an attempt to prove something to themselves and others, people of all genders may make lifestyle or social choices that are likely to lead to trouble.

An overwhelming need to belong to someone (group or individual) can colour perceptions massively. It is human to want affection and approval, no matter how hard a shell we put around ourselves. We all have a great amount of influence over each other, and this should never be underestimated. Although it can be hard for an unhappy person to recognise it, anyone who exploits the basic need for affection is not a good role model, partner or person.

The Social Group

In many ways we define ourselves by whatever group we believe we belong to. Within each of our lives, friends are a powerful force. Teenage rebellion from family values is an accepted feature of modern life. Listening to the child may help, or it may be rejected out of hand. Good friends can also be encouraged.

In many cases, friends are chosen who epitomise the opposite characteristics to those of the family, especially if the family unit is felt to be unsatisfactory. After all, 'you can't choose your family, but you can choose your friends'.

Friends may be visibly destructive and unpleasant, but they should not be condemned or banned. Parents shouldn't feel that they have 'failed' if their teenager seems to be rebelling somewhat – they have not. There are few families who do not experience a challenge from their teenage children. Of course families are composed of individuals who may have their own issues, or are struggling with uncertainties of their own.

The idea that there is another, happier way to live life may gain some leverage, however, if the parents take the time to listen to their child. Concern might be shown as to whether they are unhappy – or jealous. These parents will have more of a chance to set things right, provided the young person can find that they still care about the parent.

The issues will become even more clouded if a parent openly forbids or discourages them from associating with a certain friend, as this will only make the child less likely to view them objectively.

If your child has a friend whose actions are potentially dangerous or harmful, it is possible to enquire after them in a non-confrontational way. The possibility of their goodwill can be questioned without saying they are bad people. But anyone from the young person's chosen group of friends who appears to be genuinely caring, positive in outlook and encouraging rather than destructive might be welcomed.

Good friends can never be chosen for a child, however frustrating this may be for parents.

It is easy to lose sight of the fact that we do not deserve to be punished (physically or emotionally) by those we meet every day. Sometimes this has to be said. Seeing that there are people in our lives whose presence is not nourishing, but instead damaging, is important for the person who self harms and for their nearest and dearest. It is difficult to recognise that pain and shame are not necessary to life, however, once self harm has become a habit. While we think of this in terms of physical pain, it is no less true of emotional pain.

The individual has already become accustomed to thinking of themselves in a deeply derogatory way.

As with most aspects of thinking during self harm, the changes are not going to happen overnight. The message that self-punishment is not necessary may slowly begin to take root if it is said quietly and in an affectionate, unexaggerated way. However, pointing it out too forcefully to the unhappy person may be met with barriers.

As with most aspects of thinking during self harm, the changes are not going to happen overnight. The message that self-punishment is not necessary may slowly begin to take root if it is said quietly and in an affectionate, unexaggerated way.

In order for a better self-image to grow, time and gentle support must be freely offered.

Activity: Picture the Scene

Julie must leave her school, because her family is moving to another part of the country. Now she finds herself afraid of the new situation. She no longer feels that she is loved – or even deserves to be loved, and has started to think that the world would be better without her. Her appetite is affected, and she begins to suffer from vomiting and headaches.

She grew up with a strong group of friends and while she has always been quiet, she was also comfortable and cheerful. Now, she is afraid and nervous around her new classmates. She has no experience of establishing new friendships. Her father only really admits there is any problem, when Julie is found to be cutting herself. She wears long sleeves and hides the evidence.

Her mother doesn't know how to help, but she's worried about the changes she's noticed in her daughter.

Which groups within the new school is Julie at risk from? What might make her realise that they are a negative influence? What help is needed to stop this negative cycle? How is Julie's new environment affecting her body image? How do you think Julie is likely to respond to negative attention in school? How can Julie move to a better social environment and escape her current problems?

In Your Skin

Self-caring should always be encouraged, whenever the chance arises. Sometimes, we say that someone is "happy in their own skin", when we mean that they are happy in themselves. In the context of self harm, this becomes an even more telling phrase. The skin (and body in general) is often the first thing that someone will decide to attack if they are unhappy enough to damage themselves.

Their frustrations, sadness and anger are all taken out on their own body.

Meanwhile, people are more likely to move in a confident way and care more for their body when they become happier in themselves.

Summing Up

- Not all friends are good ones whose attentions make us feel better about ourselves. A healthy friendship is essential for all human beings.

- A friend may have become an established feature of life before it becomes clear that they are a negative influence, because friendship is by definition usually a fairly long term relationship.

- It is unlikely that you will be able to change your friend's personality, but you could try pointing out that their negative attitudes are not doing anyone any good.

- To fill the role of 'friend' in your life, you may decide that it's easier to build a new connection with someone else.

- In the next chapter, we will discuss peer groups, which are much wider than friendship groups.

- Friends are the most intimate part of our peer group.

- You can ask questions if your friend has a very negative outlook, in the hope that this will help, but without professional training you may simply find yourself more and more tangled in their negativity.

- If, after a while, you find yourself saying of someone "she makes me tired" or "I wish for once he would see the bright side", that person is a drain on your emotional resources, and beginning to be hard work.

- Some people have a real talent for draining others' energies and making people feel bad, – because of their own fears and insecurities.

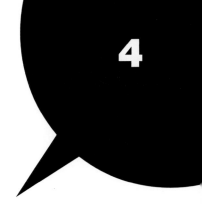

4

Peer Pressure

As with specific individual friends, peers may be positive or negative. They may inspire, or lead us into a dark view of the world which is difficult to shake. Anyone with whom you have something in common (in some way or another) can be classed as a member of your peer group. Our peers include those who share our interests, and our attitudes, values and beliefs.

Everyone who lives in the same area as you, is the same age, works at the same place or goes to the same school is your peer. Our peers also include people who relax in the same ways as us, be that through sports, music, drugs, alcohol or gaming.

Everyone's personality holds an important core of certain values, ideas and attitudes, however easy it is to believe that we don't really concern ourselves with them. The role of the peer group in this is crucial.

Our peers can either drain us or help us feel energised and enthusiastic. We can consider what they represent, and distance ourselves emotionally from anything that is unacceptable.

We do not have to share the same values, ideas and attitudes as our peers, and a major part of good mental health centres around being able to recognise that this being the case doesn't make our peers any less important to us.

We need to make certain decisions about what and who to include in the closest parts of our lives, and when we are coping with the urge to self harm it is vital that we can identify good and bad peer group pressures.

We need to make certain decisions about what and who to include in the closest parts of our lives, and when we are coping with the urge to self harm it is vital that we can identify good and bad peer group pressures.

Risk Taking

There is no doubt that excessive risk taking – which gives a 'buzz' that is pleasurable at first, has many levels. Some people are willing to take unnecessary risks with their sanity, wellbeing and body – but what causes them to do that? Well, the entirety of a body's chemical priorities change when we are afraid, as our bodies begin to release adrenaline. Without the need for or expense of illegal drugs, we are provided with a natural chemical high.

Once they have experienced the high, and addiction has begun its insidious course, they also find that they have the admiration or approval of their peers, and body chemicals are supported further by an increased sense of belonging. Serious consequences may eventually be felt, however, as more and greater thrills are required to maintain this high, and greater risks are taken. The risks that individuals take at this point are no less self-harming than actually sitting down and cutting.

It is the encouragement and teasing of the peer group that urges someone to take the first few risks, even though at the beginning, the individuals are more likely to feel scared than thrilled.

The individual who is basically less confident may deal with this in a number of ways. Peer group approval can sometimes feel just as addictive as the rush itself if the individual was initially uncertain or awkward (even if they were hiding this well).

Individuals with Lower Confidence

If the self-harm comes in the form of excessive risk-taking, the individual may present as someone who is devil-may-care and enjoys a degree of confidence and bravado. Risk taking can however become addictive, and even if it does not, it can lead individuals into some very dangerous places. Such individuals are particularly difficult to help, since they take a great deal of pride in the image that they project to the world.

If the personality traits we might more readily associate with self-damage are present in an individual, they may be more at risk than others of developing these risk-taking behaviours. Their personal uncertainties may lead them straight to despair, and to self-harm, or they may seek the approval of a peer group or other negative relationship, which will also lead to self-harm through risk taking.

Some people who are less confident will become a bully in order to cover their insecurities, while others may find they attract the attention of the bullies discussed in Chapter Three. Each of these individuals lacks a full sense of their own self-worth, and usually suffers massive anxieties, which they hide from the rest of the world. Common ground is shared by each of these individual types.

Parents – who 'only want the best' for their children will often confuse 'the best' with 'being the best achiever'. Parents also often believe that they are doing the right thing by their children, by making attempts to 'toughen them up'. Another kind of parent may over-protect their child, and never truly let them develop their own coping mechanisms. Excessive expectations from parents can sometimes add to these self-doubts and anxieties. Any support which argues against their negative self-belief will help.

The concept of 'meaningful occupation' is worth considering, here. A child who is happy and secure in their own limits is much less at risk of self harm and has been given the greatest gift of all by his parents – after all, very few of us are actually destined to be Nobel Prize winners or award-winning actors. Prestige and prosperity are not necessary for a goal or occupation to be worthwhile.

A meaningful occupation may bring no financial reward at all, but carries the reward of making us believe that we – and our lives – have some meaning.

'Niall' had high expectations for his son, and didn't realise that they were damaging. *'I'm okay about him being a graphic designer –'* He was alright with his son's choice of career, and was proud that he was being so relaxed about it. But he always clarified his statements with the line, *'so long as he's good enough to become a world-famous graphic designer!'*

A realistic expectation can go a long way.

We define ourselves by our activities, so what's most important is that we are able to find something we enjoy and feel good about.

Children are best equipped to deal with the world and its problems if their self-confidence is nurtured and allowed to develop. They don't need to be toughened up, they need to be encouraged.

When there are crises and difficulties, some parents have a tendency to blame themselves, instead of putting their energies into support and problem solving. There is no one in the world who always gets parenting right – parents must walk a fine line at all times.

The best kind of parent provides guidance and boundaries as well as love for their child. In a situation where if the child breaks the law or exceeds social boundaries, he or she understands that there are consequences, and must face them. A child's mental health can actually be damaged by unnecessary sheltering from a parent. The phrase 'tough love' is sometimes used to describe the more balanced form of parenting.

How we deal with difficult times or personal uncertainties depends very much upon the emotional habits that we have learned. We are all haunted by demons at sometimes, ideas that lurk in the darkest corners of our minds. We can learn good habits that allow us to take control of our demons, though. A habit is just a habit, and if it is bad, negative or counter-productive, it can always be replaced.

I Need to Be Liked

One of the bully's most cruel and destructive tools is to make someone believe that no one likes them. Feeling liked is important to all of us in some way or another. The entire human race share this same fear as the individual who self harms, it just isn't so immediately obvious. While someone whose self-image suffers in this way may be helped by counselling, there is also a school of thought that warns us that too much analysis and introspection may be counter-productive, for some individuals.

We all have an 'inner child', a powerful part of our personality, who is going to influence our response to trouble or stress. The inner child badly needs to know that they are liked, which is different from being told that they are loved. (Psychologists call this 'unconditional positive regard'.) Even with help, anxieties about being hated, not accepted or disliked are usually deeply entrenched, and are not going to vanish overnight.

Sometimes, the most help can come from a friend who simply remains cheerful and encourages happy, non-threatening activities, over a length of time. We can begin to see how to help an unhappy person grow if we think of them as someone whose inner child is afraid, more often than laughing.

Love becomes a complex – difficult to resolve – issue in the mind, and may even be rejected as a concept completely. Love is not real if it demands success or prestige in return for the relationship. Knowing that you are liked exactly as you are is vital for a happy inner child. Self confidence can only begin to increase if this basis is provided. If these characteristics seem to be unobtainable, it is good to 'role play' them.

Real Acceptance

Individuals who are unhappy in themselves will strive to be accepted, and may make the wrong, self-destructive decisions in order to find a sense of belonging. The other side of needing to be liked is the need to be accepted within a group. This is why it's so important to decide what might be the right reasons for being accepted, by consciously examining life and its goals.

Striving to be accepted socially for good reasons can sometimes involve making a conscious decision to adopt characteristics that are good and universally admired. These characteristics can eventually become normal behaviour after a period of role-playing, and this sort of training can bring about remarkable results.

This sort of activity can bring about changes that some people may dislike. It's possible that one or two people will be uncomfortable with you becoming a happier, healthier person. If this happens, it's worth stepping back and taking a close look at your relationship with this individual. If they do not like the changes in you that are for the better, it is time to let them go.

It's likely that they have huge issues of their own, and as a result are jealous, anxious or angry. Nourishment is more important than punishment, though, so it may be time to move on to a better, healthier relationship.

Activity

Give some thought to the idea of a 'meaningful occupation' and how you feel about it. There is no doubt that these include finding a way to describe yourself. It may include voluntary work, or something creative or simply active. The occupation can include anything that gives you a sense of satisfaction and achievement, and does not have to be paid work.

It is important to allow time to reflect on what might work as a 'meaningful occupation' to you. What makes this sort of occupation meaningful are the positives it brings. What positives would your meaningful occupation bring? It might bring the chance of new friends, the ability to say 'I am a swimmer/writer/carpenter/dancer etc.' or something to occupy your brain, and give you a strong sense of self-image.

Think about the benefits that you can expect from your choice. You can begin to pursue this activity as soon as you allow yourself to discover what this would be, by thinking of ways forward.

Summing Up

- Our lives can be strongly influenced by our peer groups.

- The influence of the peer group can never truly be separated from an individual who has begun to self harm – or who is tempted by it, either as an experiment or as an emotional statement.

- The insights that can carry an individual towards positive attitudes and better mental health are the most helpful and productive, as these will allow them to move forward.

- If we haven't had the exact same experiences as the individual, we lack the power of an insight personally gained, and our advice may not always be as useful as we think it is.

- The best action is just to be there, and to let the self-harmer know that you are listening.

- The rest of us can only offer support.

- It is important therefore to examine the individual within the wider social context of their life, and also to encourage him to do so for himself.

- 'You must talk to someone' is an acceptable approach.

- When we come to adult life, we may be said to be anti-social. Even those of us who avoid social interaction as much as possible, and convince themselves that they 'don't need people' are influenced by those around who may be counted as peers.

- There is no doubt that at some times in life many of us just want to be part of the world around us.

5

Difficult Children

U nfortunately, children and teenagers are often labelled 'difficult' when they misbehave, and while this label may be accurate, it is in itself a block to looking any further into the issues.

Education

When a young person begins to self harm, the popular psychology quote 'all behaviour is communication' becomes particularly true. Younger children who behave in non-standard ways are often described as 'difficult', and teenagers as 'rebellious' or 'surly'. This behaviour is often caused by a variety of factors, and it's always worth trying to discover what those factors are.

If someone (of any age) is behaving in a way that is troublesome or less than sociable, we should at least wonder why. We imply that there is simply no hope of any growth or development when we dismiss behaviours by saying 'they've always been difficult'. This implies that this is an inherent part of who they are, and something that can't be changed. Someone with this label who is anxious, worried, afraid, tired, just having a bad day or suddenly has big concerns on his mind will only be seen as their 'difficult' label, and other potential problems will never be addressed.

There is every possibility that a child's reputation will continue throughout school life once they are labelled as 'difficult' in school.

If a teacher is to succeed in their relationship with a child, they must stand in loco parentis (in place of the parent) while children are at school, and must appear to be the adult in the relationship. Many teachers feel shy of facing this part of their job, since they have 'far too much work' to take on any additional depth within their role. Under Section 90 and 91 of the Education and Inspections Act 2006, teachers have statutory authority to discipline pupils whose behaviour is unacceptable, who break the school rules or fail to follow a reasonable instruction (DfE, 2016). They are not required to replace parental roles and guidance – a mistake often made by those who misunderstand the phrase 'in loco parentis'. They are instead required to maintain and set boundaries, and be the adult in any situation they are in.

Children want to know where the boundaries lie, and what we often perceive as difficult behaviour is often just them trying to push the adult to see how far they are allowed to go. Something that we want may feel pretty compelling.

How does the question of boundary setting work within peer relationships? We were born to be social creatures, and this means that there are rules and boundaries. When we consider people who intentionally harm themselves, the question of boundaries and boundary setting is central to the discussion. Life is given form by the boundaries surrounding it, which can also be a source of reassurance.

Other boundaries may be so restrictive that they never allow us to grow and develop. If the boundaries of our lives change constantly and can't be relied on, despair is likely to follow. It is a short step from here to feeling worthless and unlovable, and to begin to consider self-harming activities. It can be difficult for anyone else to understand the self-harmer's feelings and reasons, but if this fact can be understood, we can begin to help.

In our dealings with other human beings, we are always walking a fine line between too many and too few boundaries. The most damaging self-image that anyone can have is perhaps to be shy and isolated, and to believe yourself to be unlikable. Many people do this. While it can be difficult to say why, such a person may carry with them a vibe of uncertainty.

With Others

People may find it difficult to fully relax around someone who does not perceive themselves to be part of a group, and they may easily gain the reputation of being a 'difficult' person. There are many potential outfalls in this development. Because this is often not consciously expressed, the attitude of his peers will also have a subtle – perhaps unconscious – effect on his own psychology and self-image.

The lonely individual may be seen as a 'loner', without his loneliness and potential despair ever being recognised. Trusting this person will come less naturally to those around them. This leads to the quick development of a vicious and self-perpetuating cycle. And although it is rapid to establish, because we are human, with human fears and insecurities, it is a hard mental habit to break.

The individual may begin to attract the wrong group of friends, whose priority is to cause others trouble and who have issues of their own that need to be dealt with. The less-than-comfortable individual may also attract the bullies discussed earlier.

We know when people treat us in certain ways, and we understand without anything being said, if they have beliefs about us. Often unwittingly, people will respond in a way that confirms an individual's own negative self-image, as it will colour every interaction they have. Yet another vicious and harmful cycle forms around the individual's negative self-image.

Self harm often has at its core a range of negative beliefs and feelings.

We are always capable of changing our self-image, but it can be difficult to do this without active support from at least one other person. It is possible to improve or change even the most entrenched negative mindset.

The Family

Siblings are notoriously jealous of each other at different times, and a great deal of hidden bullying goes on with families, which can set the stage for severe insecurities in later life. Such activities are often subtle, carefully hidden from adult observation, and have long been accepted by the other children. When it comes to the creation of a person's self-image, parents and family have a huge responsibility.

We are always capable of changing our self-image, but it can be difficult to do this without active support from at least one other person. It is possible to improve or change even the most entrenched negative mindset.

You may well benefit from a close inspection of your own attitudes if you think you are somehow the perfect parent or partner – after all, nobody on earth gets to hold this title. It is always worth pausing to observe family members. The ways in which the different children in a family actually treat each other may be the first thing that parents should try to be vigilant about.

Often, one child will be actively unpleasant (either verbally or physically) to one or more of the others, and this may come as a surprise to their parents.

A child on the receiving end of 'in-house' bullying may assume that the parent knows about it, and the implication must be that they concur and do not care. So if one of the children is becoming withdrawn, fretful and negative, it is the parent's job to discover what has led to this, and to set boundaries for the family that will stop the destructive behaviour.

Destructive things may well be happening in your home without you realising it, and observation may reveal these. While your children may think you know about everything that goes on in your home and are simply choosing not to act, they may actually be doing things that you know nothing about.

Activity: Picture the Scene

Give some thought to your own early years. Nobody's childhood is perfect, so don't be shocked if it isn't all happy memories! For the purpose of this exercise, make a list of the positives that you took away from your childhood and disregard the negatives.

- Picture a different childhood for yourself. Think about parents who are addicts, alcoholics, or severely depressed. Imagine that you, as a child, become aware that one of your parents is self harming.

- Now decide what you might need to do need to do, to undo the psychological damage that this unhappy experience causes.

- How might this affect your self belief, values, thoughts and attitudes?

This may take some time – give it as much thought as you need.

Summing Up

- It is an accepted fact that all children are a little difficult sometimes.

- This is not unnatural, but is simply part of the child's growth and development, in that he or she is trying to become an individual in their own right.

- We can help these children to change negative or destructive habits. Labelling them as 'difficult' is not helpful, unless we are clear that it is a temporary situation.

- Although the individual may be deeply unhappy, and may also feel unlovable and isolated, this is not necessarily a sign of mental illness.

6

Mental Health Issues

Early Adulthood and Adolescence

ndividuals are most likely to engage in self harm, negative lifestyle choices and serious risk taking when they are young adults and teenagers. Many people suffer at least one phase of sub-clinical (that is, not necessarily in need of medical attention) during their teenage years. Left unaddressed, chronic unhappiness can develop into actual mental health problems, so these feelings should never be discounted as passing phases. These will recur, because they have not been dealt with, and when they do, a precedent has been set by both parties.

Adolescence and early adulthood are also key times for the appearance of schizophrenia, which does need medical attention.

Pregnancy also causes huge hormonal changes, which must revert to a previous state very quickly after giving birth. It may be that the lowering of mood is never fully recognised by those around. Blue spells may recur, or may only happen very occasionally.

Doctors and psychologists describe depression as 'reactive', in that it occurs in response to something. Once the triggers are identified, it is usually possible to alter lifestyle, so that the person can grow and develop.

The psyche can really be thrown into havoc during adolescence – the body is changing a great deal, and new hormones are taking over. We must never underestimate the power of hormonal activity and change.

Non-reactive, or 'endogenous', depression is something that hasn't been accepted as a possibility for some years. The implication was that nothing could be done about this condition because the individual's personality was basically depressive, and prescription medication was the only solution. But to take this view is to completely miss the point.

If we explore the issues fully, though, we now know that something can be identified as the trigger. No one should be left on anti-depressant medication (which is largely highly addictive) for an extended length of time.

There are pitfalls to medications, but doctors may offer them to help someone over an acute episode of depression. It is necessary for the patient to reach a calmer state of mind so that they can fully engage with counselling and explore their issues in depth.

Visual hallucinations may be 'flashbacks' to the experience of drug use. The person will not have taken any substance, in order to experience the flashback. Schizophrenia isn't the only possible cause for hallucinations and similar symptoms, and it's important to remember this. A flashback is an episode that may occur without any external stimulus, causing the person to relive or intensely remember a previous experience. It is easy to miss this possibility, as an individual's drug, alcohol or substance history may not be known to family or friends.

If someone is hearing voices that aren't there saying unpleasant things, such as describing their suffering in the most derogatory terms, this is known as an auditory hallucination. This is a symptom of schizophrenia, but it could also be an indicator of a different condition. To treat someone (chemically) for schizophrenia who does not have it, is to cause more harm than good.

What sounds like a discussion in the mind between the voice of the sufferer and other voices may occur when someone is under chronic (long-term) pressure, as the internal dialogue begins to rage. They begin to interfere with everyday functioning.

> **Doctors and psychologists describe depression as 'reactive', in that it occurs in response to something. Once the triggers are identified, it is usually possible to alter lifestyle, so that the person can grow and develop.**

Stress is quite often processed using the internal dialogue – this is natural. The voices only become more insistent and troubling if the pressures increase and become chronic. If this is happening, it is important to share the fact with someone else. The issues that worry us become unbearable at this point, and the internal pressure has crossed a line.

As these harsh internal commentators become ever more insistent and intrusive, it is not uncommon for them to begin to suggest self harm. Schizophrenia, once again, is not the only explanation for this symptom. To avoid mistakenly treating someone for a condition they do not have, all avenues should be explored by health professionals.

A Cry for Help

Anyone concerned with the topic of self-harm, either personally or professionally, should pause at this point to imagine the horror of a knife that cuts the skin. If all behaviour is communication, then to cut oneself, or put the body and long-term health at risk by any means at all is a very loud and serious form of communication. 'Attention seeking' and 'only a cry for help' are just two of the phrases that are unfortunately still used today to dismiss self harm and unsuccessful suicide attempts. This is not true.

If someone is seeking our attention to this degree or is at the point where this is the only way to express desperate and overpowering feelings, the least we can do is to listen to them, and to help them to find effective professional help and support. It is often difficult to approach anyone with the problem of self-harm. This adds to the uncertainty about what should happen next.

The listening skills that we need, in order to be useful to this individual, are discussed in chapter 8, which is aimed at health professionals, but which might also be useful to anyone involved.

There is nothing 'only' about self harm or suicide attempts, even if they are cries for help. The individual has felt the need to express their feelings by terrible and harmful means, and it's important that we listen to the despair that these actions communicate. It is an extreme thing to inflict on oneself, and isn't done without reason.

Talking to Someone – Counselling

One-to-one counselling can be very beneficial. A safe place where terrors can be expressed is sometimes the one thing that someone who self harms needs. They need to be listened to.

There are several different settings where someone in crisis may find it helpful to speak in order to see their problems more clearly.

Cognitive behavioural therapy works very well, but should only be undertaken by someone who has the appropriate training. Identifying issues and challenges that can be tackled in an achievable way can be very helpful to individuals struggling with self harm, and some therapists offer this in the form of problem-solving therapy that encourages the individual to explore their own situation.

If expressing yourself and your fears in a group setting sounds like it could be helpful, group therapy may be available near you - these sessions normally take place on a weekly basis. If this is not the case, however, there are other possibilities.

Group therapy may be daunting at first, but is often highly successful. This is particularly true if the patient finds himself offered some time at a psychiatric day hospital. Chapter Eight will discuss these groups, run by professional facilitators, in greater detail. Sharing problems in a group does help, not least because it breaks the certainty that we are alone in our fears.

Support groups can be really helpful, and you may also be able to access self-help groups that are run by concerned (but non-professional) volunteers. They do not have fixed start and stop dates, and membership is fluid. And if the problems have their roots in drug, alcohol, substance abuse or social problems such as violence or being a single parent, there are even more.

There are many self-help groups out there, but some of the most successful and well-known examples include Alcoholics Anonymous and Gamblers Anonymous.

One helpful idea is to keep a diary, so that every day feelings can be expressed, as if they were being told to someone else. Recording these feelings as an on-line blog is not a good idea, and may attract comments or advice from destructive personalities. Someone who is struggling against the urge to self harm may find the gap between therapy sessions, which are usually scheduled for once a week, to be a little long.

A diary can fill this gap as well as provide a handy summary of the issues that have arisen during the week, ready for discussion with your therapist or group. Whenever we can, we should focus on positives, and record them in the diary. These are difficult to think of, at first, but they do exist, and this list can be added to, over time. It's best to remember to keep this diary private, however.

Support

Self-harm should never be ignored, as something that will lead to nothing. People who self-harm are roughly fifty times more likely than others to kill themselves. The idea that someone is not likely to go through with suicide if they talk about it is often discussed. The idea of suicide is often explored during a time of consideration if someone is feeling the urge to attempt it.

The individual needs to experiment with what can be 'handled' and what 'options' are available to them, and incidents of self harm may well occur at this point.

The urge to harm oneself can be overwhelming, but it tends to come in 'waves'. If help is not given to an individual who self harms, statistics suggest that one in three are likely to do it again within a year. Females tend to favour drug overdose, which of course is a less obvious form of self-harm. Men are more likely to self harm in its most traditional sense.

Paralysis, permanent scars and numbness are among the potential long term effects of cutting.

If you can learn to identify the urges before they gain full strength, it is possible to find someone or something which will help to divert the mind. A friend may not be available, but it is always possible to pick up the phone and talk to the Samaritans. There are help lines available for other national groups too, which are very helpful if they deal with issues that have led to the urge to self-harm.

The terrible promptings to hurt yourself will generally ease after a few hours, so it is possible (with support) to resist the temptation. For support between meetings, a good support group, whether it is run voluntarily or by professionals, will usually offer an emergency line for its members.

It is vital that individuals who experience the urge to self harm are able to talk to someone - anyone - about these feelings. This can help the feelings to pass, after a while. If you're calling a helpline like the Samaritans, have a false name ready if it helps to feel anonymous. Many callers like to use a false name, so the people running the phone lines will often ask, 'What should I call you?'

It's important that you feel comfortable talking things over with the volunteers, and understand that they are always willing to listen.

Before you find yourself overwhelmed by the urge to hurt yourself, it is a good idea to think about coping strategies.

When 'Liam' needed a distraction, he found that water helped. Sometimes he would take ice cubes out of the freezer, and work at trying to crush them with his bare hands. He found it helpful to go for a swim or take a (bitterly) cold shower. If he cut himself, it would be harmful and cause real pain, but these options provided a more harmless shock to the system.

'Yvonne' tried to make swimming a part of her weekly routine, echoing Liam's aim to swim as often as he could. Some days they felt that they did not want to exercise, but when they did, it always helped. Many others describe different sorts of exercise, which they found helped, but the key to success was always to make this a part of life on the good days, so that they could more easily help when emotional problems hit. These provide a sense of pleasure, and can therefore help to lift the mood.

Jogging was really helpful to 'Dan'. His sweat and the rain meant that the people he ran past didn't even notice if he cried when he ran on 'bad days'.

Endorphins, the body's natural chemicals, are released by any type of exercise. It can sometimes be especially effective, if you have a particular kind of music you enjoy, to try and exercise to that music.

'Barney' found that drawing red lines upon his skin, in a very slow and focused way, allowed him to 'mimic' the action of cutting himself. In doing this he mimed the actions of cutting, concentrating hard, but without any physical risk to himself. Instead of a sharp fountain pen, he used a soft sharpie. It brought him a sense of release.

'Amy' found that her urge to cut could sometimes be reduced if she did something creative. It allowed her to practice using sharp tools in a new, creative and non-threatening way and though a health professional involved with her was worried about her using scissors, Amy found it helpful to allow her body proximity to sharp objects.

The troubled mind needs to convince itself that these distractions will cause pain. Then it is possible to think of something else that can be substituted. It may take some concentration to find harmless replacements for physical harm because the urge is very much about putting oneself at risk, and it may not work immediately. Individuals should try to ignore the fact that these methods will provide a less dangerous pain, as it can leave them with a sense that they are foolish things to try.

The mind has a way of playing tricks that make us forget good things, and if they are recorded in black and white, we can bring them back. Self harm can bring a sense of relief, escapism or control, but it can be just as effective to search for these results by writing a diary. Record any new things you discover that help the urge to pass. It is important to minimise damage to the body, and record how we did that, although the habit may be hard to lose.

Creating a list of good things about yourself is another helpful thing you can do in the diary. This list can then provide a quick reassurance of the positives any time that it is read.

Professional Support

Professionals who find themselves faced with someone who has self-harmed should never be careless or derogatory about what is happening. There are several different types of professionals who can help us with self harm, though the first one we think of will always be the GP. The end of this book has a list of contact numbers for some great resources that are worth considering.

It's common to feel that you have failed in some way, especially if you are a parent concerned for your children or an individual concerned for your partner. This is not true.

In order for the damages and consequences of self harm to be properly assessed and treated, if you find someone in need of medical attention as a result of self harm (drugs, cutting, general debilitation), an ambulance must be called and the individual must attend accident and emergency. You mustn't waste time on unnecessary information about your own feelings when on the phone to the ambulance - it's important to remain calm and communicative. This will speed up the ambulance's arrival. Discharge home is the norm after a visit to A and E, but the patient may be kept in hospital for a night or two. The reason is usually to do with local Trust policy. The GP should be informed, and it is important to ask what support he can refer to.

Creating a list of good things about yourself is another helpful thing you can do in the diary. This list can then provide a quick reassurance of the positives any time that it is read.

Although there are other problems out there, it is a mistake to believe that self harm is any less of a crisis or less worthy of attention than any other condition, though even today there are professionals who make this mistake.

There is no one in the world who could not (given the right circumstances) be driven to self-harm, so we are particularly lacking in insight if we treat them any less seriously. This may be extended to (well-meaning) professional advice about who should be contacted, lifestyle and judgements about those who accompany the patient. An individual deserves to be treated very seriously if they are putting their life at risk - they are making a very strong statement.

The individual is likely to take any advice, body language and statements offered by a healthcare professional on board deeply and without question, so professionals would always do well to realise that they are dealing with someone in an emotionally vulnerable state and treat them with sensitivity and respect. As a professional, one should be able to deal with every situation as clearly as the last and avoid indulging in personal judgements. This is what it means to be a professional.

If someone you care about is kept in hospital for a night or two after being admitted for self harm, it doesn't mean they are any 'worse' than someone who is allowed home straight away.

On return home, support and guidance should be sought. While the family may or may not contain the root cause of the urge, the psychology of the person self-harming will impact upon all members, even before it is actually discovered. Our most valuable asset and source of support is likely the Community Mental Health Team. They can be particularly supportive if someone is found to be expressing thoughts about self-harm, particularly to the extent of suicidal thoughts, and will find a way to help even if the individual is not 'on the books' and known to the system.

Your GP may provide a referral for this team, or you can find their contact details online or in a phone book.

Activity

For this activity, we'd like you to make two lists. In one list, include everything you can think of that brings you pleasure. In many ways, the more silly the better. Try and remember to include people who help you, and be as detailed as possible.

- The second list should include possible distractions, such as those mentioned above, or some creative ideas of your own.

- Make these lists very neat and easy to read, and display them somewhere you can see them often.

- Think of the person you are most likely to turn to in a crisis, and tell them about these lists. This means that when terrible thoughts overwhelm you, they can remind you about your lists and encourage you to do things that will make you feel better.

Summing Up

- We need to prepare for bad times before they hit if we want to deal with them successfully. It's important to focus on positives and distractions when we feel that we must cause harm to ourselves.

- Trying to find a less dangerous substitute for pain and its release is a central idea. We should also force a space back into our life for the things that used to give us pleasure, and remember the positives in life.

7

Families

amily affairs almost always lie at the root of the problems that can lead to self harm. The impact of self-harm upon families can be massive. Before the self harm is discovered, and sometimes even before it begins, the individual's moods will have changed and everyone in the family will be responding to that, either consciously or subconsciously. But spouses can often realise before parents that an individual's mood has become extreme, and may well have already begun to wonder what is happening for their loved one.

For this reason, family members must see themselves as also being worthy of support, as this will allow them to respond to the situation in a way that won't make the self harm worse.

Being Tough but Fair

To show support we always aim to show someone that they are loved. For many people the desire to show love and support is tied up in an urge to protect (possibly at all costs) and to take responsibilities on to oneself. But this works only briefly.

You may or may not be familiar with the term 'tough love'. Whether you know the phrase or not, it can be difficult to know how to do it. The urge to ease the burden of the troubled individual can all too easily result in someone feeling the need to wrap the individual in cotton wool.

The roots of the individual's problems are not solved if they are not allowed to do anything about them. Every time that this mistaken support occurs, the situation is continuing and becoming more and more entrenched. The surrounding issues will come back again and again, and the individual's relatives or partner are now cast in the role of rescuer and expected to take responsibility. But it does no good, and may even harm the situation or damage the relationship.

Something that we need is a lot more basic. Tough love, based on the needs of both parties and perhaps society in general, is better. There are several key factors. Tough love is about helping the sufferer to gain firmer ground, by showing him where it can be, and how they can begin to move towards it. Boundaries are a vital part of tough love. We must show (and tell!) the individual that we love them, but that there are limits to our non-judgmental support.

For example, we can accompany them to their first counselling appointment or help the individual to arrange the meeting, but also make it clear that we can't help them if they aren't trying to help themselves. It is not acceptable to speak for the individual during their counselling session, or to insist on giving your version of events.

Love has the potential to be strong in a negative way, which is why tough, considered love is such a powerful thing.

> **Love has the potential to be strong in a negative way, which is why tough, considered love is such a powerful thing.**

Parents

Adrenaline works for us, in that it helps us to find extra energy to deal with an acute situation. But it can also produce other powerful feelings and responses, and it is important that these are understood for what they are, because some of them need to be avoided or at least curtailed. It can be extremely distressing and scary to discover that your child has begun to self harm.

The threat to a child is one of the strongest 'fight or flight' triggers imaginable, so discovering that they have hurt themselves will begin the rapid flow of adrenaline in your body.

In extreme cases, it could fall to the parents to help their child to breathe again, or to stop the bleeding.

One result of the flow of adrenaline feels natural, in that many people become angry with the person who has self-harmed. The person who has self-harmed is likely to already believe themselves to be unlovable, and will be in an emotionally fragile state. So it is best that anger is not expressed. You may well add to their beliefs about being unloved if you express your anger too freely.

Children living lives that are quite secret from their parents' is not uncommon. Many parents will feel that they are in some way inadequate if they discover their child is self-harming, and they may well feel that they have failed. A good parent tries to respond to this situation without becoming critical or judgmental. Parents must always remember that they need not be alone, either.

It can be very damaging when a parent belittles their own children, or pushes them towards extreme or unreasonable goals.

Parental responses – the result of adrenaline flow – are natural, but need to be carefully handled. When the child is ready to talk, they need to know that their parents are there to listen about their issues. For this reason, it's very important that the parent calmly stays with the child while they are treated for the damage. Creating more drama will not help anyone. Parents in this situation should seek out assistance and allow it to work. There is support available to them, as this is a sadly common issue to be dealing with.

Significant Others

Many of the responses felt by parents, described above, will also be shared by the husband, wife or partner of someone who begins to self-harm.

The most common reaction is guilt, when we discover that someone we thought we knew well has begun to self-harm. However, the likelihood is that before self-harm has become a reality, the individual has long since begun to distance himself from anyone who has been close. It is hard to believe that a relationship can survive a self-harm incident, but important to try.

Someone who goes on to self-harm has already locked themselves away in a very dark place, and has become convinced that there is no one who can help. All too often a person who self-harms but who is also in a close relationship will begin the secrecy by trying to protect their partner from their own fears and worries, but this quickly becomes a vicious circle when those fears are not expressed.

It is unlikely that a spouse who has asked questions about their partner's changing mood will receive any answers right away, and they are likely to take the changes in their partner very personally. Partners may feel that they don't actually know this person any more' – and this is particularly true if the individual has always been there for them to rely on.

There are as many reasons for this breakdown of communications as there are individuals to experience it. Uncertainty and anger prompted by an adrenaline rush are just as much an issue for spouses as they are for parents.

Spouses should talk to the GP about their fears and uncertainties, so that any help or support can be made available to them. Avoiding becoming judgmental, frustrated or critical is once again very important, as is being there to listen. Concerned family and friends also use their listening skills when offering support and it is important to be clear just what those skills are.

Both parties will struggle even more if effort is not made to keep the lines of communication open.

There will always be something or someone who can offer support to spouses in this situation, though support does vary in different parts of the country.

The Kids

Children look to us as parents to be strong and capable. Someone who has begun to self-harm is no longer a strong, capable person, and children will know this, however well hidden. It may not be immediately obvious that the child is thinking this, and after a length of time this idea can be difficult to dislodge. This is traumatic for anyone, but particularly a child, who will have a long hard struggle ahead of himself, trying to make sense of what has happened.

We should never forget that the children of someone who begins to self-harm probably need help and guidance in their own right, as they have a particular set of problems to deal with. They are not to know that a response to the world is faulty and dangerous. They need their parents to fill the role of protector and teacher, even if they don't always agree with their parents' judgement.

Kids see adults use a range of different coping mechanisms to deal with the world, and learn these behaviours from the adults around them. Discovering the body of someone whose self harm has become a successful (or nearly successful) suicide is an atrocious thing for a child, but something that is not unheard of.

Children, and especially young children, tend to believe that adults' problems are something that they have caused, whether those problems are self harm or a messy divorce. All of these issues need particular attention for the child.

'Teresa submitted her children to emotional neglect, hostility, unpredictability and confusion, and admits to having been 'an inconstant mother'. They began to pick up certain behaviours from her, and she reached a real turning point when she realised this was happening.

Play therapy, writing and artwork are successfully used to help children, and the skill of the adult professional is never to put their own (or indeed any adult) interpretation on what is being said, done or created. As with any counselling situation, it will take time for the child to trust the therapist and the situation, which can never be rushed.

Someone who specialises in dealing with children should be on hand to provide professional help and guidance and allow the child to grow through this difficult time. The child should be allowed to take their time to explain their actions and feelings in their own words.

Friends

The friends of the self-harmer will be impacted by their friend's situation - they are often deeply important to the individual, which is why we discuss them several times within this book. There are no official counselling routes to support the friend of someone who has self-harmed.

If self harm has warning signs, it's easy to think that we, as the person's friends, should have been able to spot them, and that we have failed if we didn't manage to do this. There is a limit to what we can do to help someone who is busy establishing barriers and distance, so there's no use feeling guilty about failing to prevent the inevitable. Phoning the Samaritans to talk about the experience can be beneficial while dealing with the traumatic experience, and may help clear your head so you are more capable of supporting your friend in their time of need.

Seeking Support

Different help suits different needs and situations, and it is important to accept the right kind of guidance and support. Anyone who is concerned about an individual who self-harms will be able to find professional help somewhere. How this help works is discussed elsewhere in this book, but the important thing to know is that it does exist, and it's not just for the self-harmer.

There are many among us who are involved in the help and support of those who self-harm, but who are not health professionals. The community mental health team will certainly know whatever is available in the local area, and will also know of support that relates to specific problems such as drugs, alcohol, gambling and domestic violence. Most GPs will have a range of support options to offer patients, though not every doctor will be familiar with every single possibility.

It is important to ask about support and, if the professional is unable to help, ask who can.

Activity

Could you direct someone to more information or a self-help group? If someone we know begins to self-harm, what can we do about it? Do you know how to communicate that you are here to listen to that person? How might she respond?

- Make a list of the things that you think it is most important to do.
- Think of phrases that could help here, and create a list.
- Create a third list of the things that you should avoid saying or doing.

If you needed help, how would you like to be treated? Discuss your ideas with someone else.

Summing Up

- Knowing someone who self-harms will always be an emotional point in our lives, whatever our relationship to the individual.

- We may well feel guilty, and this might be justified if there was something (for instance, bullying or abuse within the family) which we wondered about but were never brave enough to deal with.

- There is no doubt that we can, while adrenaline takes over our emotions, easily say or do the wrong thing in an already fragile situation.

- A simple hug will go a long way, or a hand held – without words – just to let the sufferer know that you are there.

- Angry words will never help any situation, so if you don't feel capable of saying something positive it is better to stay silent.

- It is important that the lessons we carry forward from these situations can become positive ones, as we learn a lot about ourselves in extreme situations.

- We may know that we are not to blame, but it can be difficult not to feel guilty. But it is still important to look at this honestly, and to resolve to be a better friend, a braver advocate and more genuinely supportive within the situation, in future.

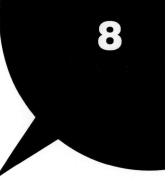

8

The Professional Point of View

This chapter contains information that can be of use to anyone, though it is mostly aimed at the health professionals themselves. Those who are involved in support groups, Samaritans and other voluntary work will also find it useful.

Activity

Take a moment to consider…

- How desperate must someone be to do this to themselves?
- What could happen that might cause you to consider self harm?
- What responses to our situation would cause you more emotional harm?
- In what way might you hurt yourself?
- What responses would you be desperate to hear if you ended up reaching this point?

Listen Up

Being listened to and being able to find a safe space in which to express feelings is crucial to regaining health. Being a good listener is therefore much more than acquiring a skill. Being a good listener is about more than just not talking. There are many people who believe that they do this well, but who in fact fall short of best practice. If someone is thinking ahead to the next question, the person being listened to will 'sense' that very quickly.

The only possible response to this is not to trust the listener, and to set a distance from them.

Maintaining eye contact (that isn't staring or threatening) and paying attention to what the individual is saying is one way to communicate that you are listening attentively and willingly. If our minds are not fully focused, our body language will almost always betray us. The listener's body language will send out subtle clues that the speaker can pick up on.

Good listeners speak as little as possible, without being actually silent, which would be intimidating. The listener's questions are not important. Actually listening fully and with full attention is the only way to communicate your willingness to listen. This means that the speaker can relax, and learn to trust the listener. It is the speaker who sets the pace and what they wish to communicate will emerge naturally, and all for the better without prompting or teasing.

If the listener does not gain the trust of the speaker, key issues will never be shared. It is alright to be silent, and while many people dislike silence, the speaker can learn that silence can also be a comfortable part of communication, and allow themselves to relax. Remember not to break the speaker's flow by interrupting them - often, it's enough to murmur or make a small noise of assent to let them know that you're still listening.

'Mirroring' is the term given to the body language that echoes the speaker's body language and posture. The skill of echoing back what the speaker has said, sometimes as a question, is known as 'reflection'. Echoing by reflection or mirroring tells the speaker that nothing he says is being judged or commented upon. These methods can let the speaker know that they are not being threatened or discounted in any way, and reassure them that they are being listened to.

If an opinion is asked, the response should always be to say that it is the speaker's opinion and feelings that matter. Opinions on what is being said do not need to be offered by the listener. Encouraging the speaker to see their opinion as important can result in better insight and understanding, as they can then be encouraged to explore their feelings further.

Those who self-harm have been badly lacking a feeling of achievement in their lives, but when they are listened to by a good listener the insights that are achieved also bring a sense of achievement.

You may well be saving a life, just by listening to someone properly.

Facilitating a Group

Best practice in group work, which is known as facilitation, is for two professional leaders to work with the group. It should always be remembered that if one-to-one counselling can be scary enough, and will always take time to relax into, the presence of others, probably strangers, must be even more so. There are several situations where group work might be offered.

Several other people who may or may not share the same problems or similar ones will often be encouraged to carry out group work together. Certain groups aim to address a particular type of issue and run for a set number of weeks. They have a start date and must run their course without anyone new being added to the membership. If a date is set for a group to start, and it runs for six weeks, then someone who presents with similar problems after it has started cannot join and gain the benefit for quite some time.

Those who self-harm have been badly lacking a feeling of achievement in their lives, but when they are listened to by a good listener the insights that are achieved also bring a sense of achievement.

They may well (subliminally) feel further marginalised or discounted.

These are known as 'closed' groups. This approach has a few obvious problems. The support that the group might offer could end up being withheld if someone seeks support after the group has started, and they will have to wait and cope without support until another group is run.

'Open' groups are also run, however. At these groups, newcomers are only asked to introduce themselves at first and to listen. They can join the group at any stage and stay as long as they like, as the system is more fluid.

Tensions develop sometimes within the group, and each of the facilitators should always be aware of these. Facilitators should always be careful to avoid creating an 'us and them' situation, and should not sit next to each other for this reason. This helps to avoid the sense that this is in any way a lecture or a lesson by preventing the professionals from dominating the flow of the group and allowing the focus of the group to range around the room.

The facilitators must practice keeping their body language open, non-judgmental and genuinely friendly. To keep the balance of the conversation flowing, both facilitators have equal status and may interject with prompts like 'Is that what you were describing the other week, Julie?' or 'Let's let Mark finish talking before moving on.'

About ten minutes before the end of the session, one of the facilitators (preferably not the same one each week) should mention the time, and that the session is coming to a close. All concerned should know when the session is going to end, and a group that lasts more than an hour is unlikely to prove beneficial. Just as in one-to-one work, timing can make a big difference to group sessions.

If someone makes a habit of being late, they are trying to draw attention to themselves in some way – perhaps which cannot comfortably be discussed in the group. Members should be encouraged to be on time so that group sessions can begin promptly. Try to discuss the lateness of certain members with the individuals on a one-to-one basis so as not to distract the group from its goal.

Sometimes a gently, achievable target may be set for the next week. The group as a whole should always be thanked at the end of the session, and particular contributions may be mentioned. It is important to say 'thank you' and 'well done' to anyone who has spoken in a significant way. It should be made clear that individuals can speak to the facilitators privately if there is something troubling them, and all members should get to leave with a sense of achievement.

Activity

If you are a health professional, try to ask yourself these questions on a regular basis.

- Can I find a calm stillness within myself, which I can call upon so that I act gently and professionally in a difficult situation?

- Can you use this so that everyone (patient, relatives and professional team alike) learn from the experience?

- Is anyone around likely to interfere with my efforts to calm the situation, and if so can they be delegated to deal with some other aspect of the situation?

- What can we all learn from how we operated?

- What do I understand by open questions?

- What does the term 'listening skills' mean to me?

- What is the best way to deal with a situation in a way that will calm the sufferer if I believe I can only spare them a certain amount of time?

- Can I avoid language that suggests prejudice or judgement when I document these discussions? (Keep in mind that the words you include in medical records are considered a legal document.)

- After the discussion, will we have time to debrief and make notes?

- In what way do you use your tone of voice, words and body language? Imagine yourself to be the team leader, and consider what guidance you would give to someone less experienced than yourself to help them.

Activity: Picture the Scene

Give some thought to the people in your caseload (if you are a medical professional). You have the potential for a group if you can identify things that some of your patients have in common. You may already have your group if you are part of a voluntary support network. Before you begin, however there are certain questions to be asked.

- How will you explain the group to potential members, and what might you say to persuade them to join?

- What might follow?

- What are the rules and boundaries?
- How often will you meet? Where?
- What protocols might you want to put in place?
- And what is the optimum number of members, excluding yourself and your co-facilitator?
- Who can you rely upon to co-facilitate with you?
- What does this group hope to achieve?
- Is it something specific or more general?
- Do you and your co-facilitator disagree on any points?
- Will your group be mixed or single-sex?
- Will people be able to join at any point, or will it be a closed programme?
- Will you keep a record of the discussions?

The group will not founder within a few weeks if you are able to answer these questions before you begin, as this means that structure is in place and you are ready to resolve any issues.

Summing Up

- In any situation, these approaches can provide the basis of good practice in helping those who self-harm.

- Always remember to allow the individual to make progress at their own pace.

- The saying 'pain is what the patient says it is' holds very true in health practice.

- The individual who is self-harming is the only person who can judge when things are getting better, and those providing support should believe that it hurts when the patient says it does.

- The individuality of the individual is key.

- While the individual will find himself listened to, and regarded, he will learn that he is not under pressure to perform in any way.

9

Loving Yourself

Human self-esteem is a very fragile thing, and may be a construct that is built upon the flimsiest of foundations. Self-esteem is a major issue for anyone who self-harms. A very insecure personality may sometimes be disguised, however, by a carefully crafted front.

Anything that potentially threatens human life can be considered a form of self-harm and in many ways a cry for help, however well-hidden, and there is no doubt that excessive risk-taking falls into this category. Substance use is again a case in point.

It is vital that the growth of good self-esteem is addressed, as a person's mental health strongly hinges on their opinion of themselves.

Needs and Wants

We will discuss Maslow's Hierarchy of Needs in a moment. Before we can recognise the role that they play in our mental health, we need to understand how different wants and needs are from each other, and how important these differences are. The real main difference between these two is that a want can be counter-productive, in our mental health, causing us to have a very skewed view of the world, and our place within it.

If we have no hope of gaining what we want, we may waste an incredible amount of time – years, even – daydreaming about the possibility. Obviously to be this preoccupied with something we want is far from healthy, and there may come a time when we have to face that we need to step back from this obsession. For many, all energies and ideas are taken up with trying to gain what they want, and there's no doubt that wants can become the focus of our life.

An obsession can easily develop around the things that we want. But this is an unrealistic way to define ourselves, and something we must work to avoid.

Even if we don't really need something, a want can begin to feel like a need if we let it get out of hand. We should instead be working towards our actual needs as these (as outlined by Abraham Maslow in 1943) are things that can support us in our mental health. This is the true definition of a need – not just something we want very, very badly.

Physiological needs include air, water, food and sleep. Safety is also a basic. Safety needs and physiological needs are among the first on Maslow's list of needs. It is also here that we can see possible things to focus on, to bring us back to mental health. It can also be a very useful tool, helping to guide individuals away from self-dislike and towards acceptance of self, and a happier, fuller life.

> **We must always address physiological needs first, as mental health is impossible without them. Mental health is also going to suffer if we are unable to feel safe and secure in our surroundings.**

We must always address physiological needs first, as mental health is impossible without them. Mental health is also going to suffer if we are unable to feel safe and secure in our surroundings. Although necessary to mental health, we can often lose sight of our self esteem and the ways in which we define ourselves if we fail to look at wants and their relationship to needs (as defined by Maslow).

Defining a "need" is not the only thing that Maslow's Hierarchy of Needs does.

What Do We Need?

This is a key question, in the context of self harm. Several other writers have argued that basic needs cannot be structured into a hierarchy. Maslow famously wrote that he studied healthy human beings to arrive at his model, because 'the study of crippled, stunted, immature, and unhealthy specimens can yield only a cripple psychology and a cripple philosophy'. He included such figures as Albert Einstein and Eleanor Roosevelt in his study, as well as a group of very high scoring students.

A triangle is normally used to represent Maslow's Hierarchy of Needs. Our very basic physical and safety needs must be in place before we can hope to maintain (or return to) mental health. Some of Maslow's critics would argue that safety needs are just as basic as physiological needs, and there is no doubt that in terms of mental health and well-being, they are very close.

Rather than just labelling them negatively, Maslow's aim was to help those in crisis return to mental health. In terms of good mental health, it could be argued that noteworthy figures like Einstein are not really representative of the general population, but it could also be argued that Maslow's studies aimed to describe how we could all reach their level of success. But it is important to remember that probably more than half of these people were regarded as eccentric.

When trying to help individuals find their way back to their life purpose and self, Maslow's is a good model. It can really come in handy for those who need to regain their sense of self.

Physical Needs

The following essential, basic physical needs all appear on Maslow's list:

- **Health.** An individual needs to be in a state of complete emotional and physical well-being in order to be deemed "healthy". This optimal state of health can only be maintained if the individual has access to proper healthcare.

- **Water.** It is a basic human right that everyone should have access to safe water, as it is a fundamental human need. The physical and social health of all individuals is jeopardised if water is contaminated. Human dignity is also affected if this right is removed. Clean water is a luxury that remains out of the reach of many, even today. Nearly two and a half billion live without basic sanitation worldwide, while more than a billion have no access to improved water sources. It is no coincidence that these people rank among the least healthy and poorest in the world.

- **Clothes.** The human need for clothing is just part of our need for an adequate standard of living. In fact, acute poverty is often signalled if someone is ill-clothed. The poor, including the unemployed, under-employed and working poor are among those who suffer most from a lack of adequate clothing. As Dr Stephen James explains in A Forgotten Right?: The Right to Clothing in International Law:

  > "We see it in the shivering or sweltering discomfort of 'beggars,' the homeless, the drug dependent and the 'derelict,' the elderly, the invalided, the 'street kid' or the just plain poor. Their plight has provoked condemnation, blame, disgust and derision, but religious, moral and secular creeds have in contrast exhorted us to respond with love, charity, mercy, with empathy and in a spirit of justice."

- **Sex** is listed as a basic need, but its position in the hierarchy is ambivalent, since it is also included in other levels of the triangle. Love and belonging is the most notable of these. But sex can be included in all levels of the hierarchy, to a greater or lesser degree. How much of a need sex is at different levels is a very individual thing, but should never be underestimated.

- **Food.** Reasonable nutrition, rather than just quantity. A hungry person cannot focus on improving his mental health. That need has to be met first. But poor diet can affect us much more deeply than simply causing hunger. Diet is about healthy eating – not diet regimes and a good diet is one that includes fruit, vegetables, meat or other protein and keeps fats, sugars, high-carb snacks, alcohol and fry-ups to a minimum.

  > The argument runs that a person's mental health cannot be successfully improved, if he or she remains hungry. The body has too much to struggle for, before it can allow energy to be expended upon regaining mental health. This argument can extend to bad nutrition, such as too much caffeine, junk food and so on, all of which can adversely affect the mental state, if taken in large amounts.

Security

This is where – for many people – a need for a fairly ordered life, and the sense that they are in control of what happens to them, comes strongly into play. Our safety needs are the next most important, once our basic physiological needs are met. It could also be argued that our safety needs are no less basic or essential than our physiological.

For some people, of course, a well-ordered life would be an unpleasant thought as they enjoy a sense of risk in life. Trying increasingly dangerous practices can, however, put both mental and physical health at risk.

We should take the time to ask ourselves why putting oneself at risk appeals to some individuals. While a person may see these thrills as part of what gives life meaning, they may also risk losing life, eventually. The psychology behind this may be rooted (for some) in a need to punish oneself. An increasing wish to approach a real danger point is, as we have seen, common among those who self-harm.

Danger and pain can also become an addiction for some individuals.

Personal Security

How far is the individual's life at risk? Are other people a threat or an incentive? At this point in Maslow's list, our attention turns to personal safety. If there are any risks present, what are the causes? Mental health, certainly, cannot hope to improve for those living in a 'risk' situation.

Money

The real point about financial security is that a person believes they are secure. It is hard to live in our world without worrying about money, but it is important to recognise that those worries can be greatly over-exercised. Once again, the answer lies within self-perception, and learning to feel okay inside.

Different individuals believe in different ways to financial security. Whatever the course adopted, there is no doubt that most people in our society are forever struggling towards something more, in terms of finances.

Many of us dream about financial security - it's something most of us strive for. Some people are forced to resort to crime to achieve financial security, while others are able to reach it through their career. Some people dream of fame and fortune, or of winning the lottery. Money problems are not overwhelming for everyone, of course: A select few are genuinely unconcerned by finances and live on the edge of society quite happily.

For some, good mental health becomes unattainable because they have developed an obsession with money. There is no amount of money in the world that can make someone feel safe once the feeling of insecurity has taken hold.

Health and Well-Being

What on earth does this mean? As I once heard someone say to a doctor who was prescribing anti-depressants rather than looking at physical symptoms, 'If you felt as ill as I do, you'd feel depressed too'. These will be discussed further in chapter 12 (good health and its promotion), but for now it is important to see that a sense of good health must be included in the safety needs.

If someone is suffering from a long-term illness, they will eventually begin to feel trapped by it, and may come to resent the loss of the life they once knew. Whether or not we are physically healthy can make a big difference. The health and abilities we once took for granted can slowly disappear as we age, and many people feel angry about that loss.

Spiritual, emotional, social and physical attributes are all combined to create a whole person, and in health care these days we tend towards a **holistic** view of people where we aim to treat the whole person.

Mental health can create a vicious circle in individuals who appear to suffer constant ill health, and who worry about all sorts of serious illnesses, as they have moved into a serious, unhealthy preoccupation.

Belonging and Affection

This is the third level in Maslow's hierarchy of needs. Good mental health is not attainable for individuals who suffer from the belief that they are not loved, and that they can never fit into everyday life. But sometimes – especially during adolescence – young people lose a sense of their own self-worth, and believe themselves to be unlovable outsiders.

We have already said in an earlier chapter that one of the key factors for individuals are that they appear to have no close friend. When we consider people who self-harm, this becomes particularly important.

Parents may well have always met a child's safety and physiological needs, but this is not enough if the child does not receive enough love or affection. In the context of Maslow's model, it is important to recognise that this need must be addressed, so that the individual can move on, back towards mental health.

We have already discussed this issue to some extent in an earlier chapter.

Esteem

There is no doubt that the sense of love and belonging, which was lacking in the previous stage, is a question of perception. We are ready to move on to the next level of need once the need to feel loved and lovable is addressed. To achieve his esteem needs, he must allow himself to believe that he has love and a group of people to belong to. Some exercises that can help with this are discussed later.

Both self-esteem and the esteem of others fall under the need for esteem. Other people may well love, respect, admire and draw inspiration from an individual. But if the individual is unable to perceive that this is the case, they cannot benefit from this affection. Not a bit of it. Only once this is accepted can the individual's self-esteem be improved.

In this way he can begin to develop the necessary self-esteem, by discovering more about himself, and by giving himself credit for his good points. By living in this way, they could be said to epitomise good mental health.

Listening is a great tool for allowing someone to grow and express themselves, and is also a good way to identify signs that the individual is lacking in self-esteem. Full mental health cannot be gained until self-esteem and the esteem of others are present.

Fulfilment

Self-actualisation, a slightly strange heading, sits at the top of Maslow's triangle. Rising to life's challenges came naturally to the individuals that Maslow studied, who were all successful, energetic people who seized life by the horns. They probably suffered from dark days, like everyone else, but this did not stop them from moving on, and back into the full flow of life.

These individuals appeared to enjoy what they did, live full lives and contribute to their part of society. In terms of good mental health, we can consider this to be something that we can all aspire to. This is self-actualisation.

Sadly, in certain circumstances, the actions and energies of any of these people could have been construed and labelled negatively. But creativity per se is also the best possible way of expression, listening to self, and learning to grow. Were the individuals surveyed by Maslow mentally unwell, just because they were a little eccentric? No matter what people may have believed at the time, we would have to say no: they allowed the creative side of their nature to blossom, and if this is an eccentricity then we should all be eccentric!

Bipolar disorder and depression have been problems for many clever, creative and highly talented people throughout history.

Any creative act – however badly executed – helps to raise the mood, so someone who allows themselves the opportunity to create, dance, exercise or help the world in some way is doing themselves a lot of good. Self-esteem for many people hinges on their ability to create something that they can be proud of.

Activity: Picture the Scene

The things that Ellie used to enjoy have all lost their appeal recently - she has been lacking in energy for a while, and has lost interest in her friends. Nobody knows that she has started cutting herself. She is beginning to cut deeper and deeper. She was shocked by the pain at first, but feels she is better at handling it now. One day, her family has to call an ambulance when she is found bleeding from a serious cut.

- Who will Ellie have to talk to?

- Will someone listen?

- How open will she be?

- What would be a good, positive thing to draw her attention to, about herself?

- How might her parents react? What are they feeling?

Summing Up

- If a person is struggling, we need to work to help them return to good health. In this chapter, we have looked at the needs that are essential to the development of good mental health.

- Before we can grow emotionally, we have certain needs that must be met. Maslow's hierarchy is shown here as it demonstrates these needs step-by-step.

- Any one of us has the potential to be a happy, creative, energetic person.

- Each step of Maslow's triangle builds securely on the last, allowing us to move up through the levels and back towards full mental health.

- What we need to learn is how to accept certain good things about ourselves.

- The image of the self-actualised individual is one that we should hold on to.

- We recognise that there are ways forward, but in times of trouble it can be difficult to see what those ways are.

10

Good Health and Its Promotion

How Do We Stay Healthy?

When we begin to look at health in general, we quickly become aware that mental and physical health are closely intertwined. Although ill-health may be evident, good health can mean different things to different people. The question 'what keeps us well?' is therefore much more difficult to answer than we might at first imagine. This does not mean that the question should not be faced.

What does feeling 'well' entail? A person who insists that "I have my health, so I don't need to change anything' may well appear to the rest of us as overweight, a smoker who struggles to breathe or an anaemic person who's worryingly pale.

Our physical health can easily have an impact on our mood, while our attitude can quickly shape our physical health. Health is more than the absence of disease. Most people would agree on a set few guidelines that would determine whether or not someone is "healthy", though many will find it easier to apply these guidelines to other people than to their own lives.

Attention to any problems that arise is vital if we want to stay healthy, and so are a good diet, exercise and fresh air. The trick is to try something, even if only for five minutes a day, building up times over an extended period.

The habit of bad eating is difficult to break, but as 'Shona' remarked – 'There is no food or drink that I want more than I want to be healthy again'.

From an early age, many of us are conditioned to believe that junk foods that offer no nutritional value are a 'reward' or a 'treat', while vegetables and healthier foods are more like taxes imposed on us by our parents. Parents believe that they are acting in the child's best interests, but in fact they can be doing untold damage.

We do know what the bad things are within our diet and lifestyle. Fresh air may be difficult in the middle of a city, but walking or visiting the park is still better than never going out, or always driving. The aim is always to increase this but again, if it can become routine and regular, this small achievable amount will work wonders.

Many of us also find exercise to be a daunting prospect. Rather than an occasional 'blast', it's often easier to make ourselves exercise if we can introduce it as a regular part of our daily routine. Unless we have a disability or condition that prevents us from doing it, we should all aim to walk or roll at least a hundred yards every day, even if the conditions are not ideal.

Many people ignore problems, because they believe they know what the doctor will say if they approach him. It is essential, above all else, that we give the necessary attention to any problems that arise. Getting a doctor's opinion may well save your life if the symptoms you've identified as "no big deal" turn out to be important.

We harm ourselves – and shorten our lives – by failing to make necessary changes. The small changes that you need to make will take little to no effort, but many of us will still fail to make them. The impetus to change these habits must always come from the individual themselves, but it's easy to brush this off by claiming that "I can't do that; I've no willpower."

Good – or improved – physical health will lead to improved mental health, and should always be attempted, when we want to move away from self-destructive mental habits. Our state of mind really hinges on how we treat our physical body.

More about Exercise

Whenever we exercise a number of things happen. Joints keep working longer, weight remains at a healthier level, organs and systems work better, for longer. This means that each of these areas is benefitting every time we exercise. Adrenaline is released by the body, which allows more activity to take place. A little exercise is good for the body – everybody knows that!

What not everybody realises, though, is that physical activity can also have a big impact on mental health. Endorphins are released when we exercise.

In order to carry more oxygen to the muscles and brains, we begin to breathe more when we exercise. It may also help to do activities like yoga that gently focus upon breathing patterns if exercise is too difficult right now. There is no one to compete against, except ourselves, and every few days we should aim to increase what we do.

When we despair of life and need to completely revise our self-image, it is difficult to know where to start. Adrenaline has a positive beneficial effect upon attitudes, feelings and self-image. They occur naturally as a result of exercise, and although we may feel the discomfort of aching muscles at first, we should also allow ourselves to be aware of the pleasant tiredness that comes from having exercised.

The muscles and systems that a specific exercise involves aren't the only parts of your body that benefit from the exercise – each activity kicks off a positive cycle that affects your whole body. What's more, somebody who exercises can begin to enjoy new and re-remembered aspects of themselves each time they exercise – although the benefits of adrenaline are only brief, once they have been experienced, the individual will know that they can experience them again.

The body's "pleasure" chemicals, or endorphins, are a big part of exercise. If we are able to focus on the pleasure they bring us, we will be able to start new, positive mental habits that will make exercising easier in the future.

The kick start we need when we're trying to figure out how to change our lives can be found through exercise and the natural chemical responses it creates in our bodies. All concerned must continue to believe that this can be achieved, even though it looks daunting – and perhaps impossible – at first. Certainly if the endorphins described above can be brought into play, we will begin to feel better about ourselves.

Even if we don't plan to increase our exercise to become a major part of our lives, and even if our activities remain gentle, introducing a routine that involves exercise is a great way to give us a great health boost, both physical and mental.

When we despair of life and need to completely revise our self-image, it is difficult to know where to start. Adrenaline has a positive beneficial effect upon attitudes, feelings and self-image.

How Can I Improve My Mental Wellbeing?

It can be just as difficult to work on your mental health as it is your physical health. This is true even when there appears to be no real underlying pathology, but peer group pressure is actually the main factor. In the 'black hole', people can only describe themselves in terms of their relationship to others, and self-description is difficult because of the negative sense of self.

It is important to approach the problem from all possible angles. Exercise is one factor, but there are also other ways forward.

Negative beliefs and feelings are overwhelming anyone who has begun to self-harm, no matter the reason for their initial struggle. Using destructive drugs and substances may begin as a social act, but quickly lead to negative emotional changes. A certain commitment to pessimism is particularly necessary in the action of 'cutting'.

If you want to reveal something about a person's inner state, a good method is to work together in a group and begin with the question, "Who are you?" Some people may find themselves in tears from attempting to answer a seemingly simple question, as it is a deceptively difficult one for people who are struggling emotionally. Then it is important to refine the question. Those facilitating the group should smile upon any attempt at self-description and offer gentle encouragement.

"Describe yourself/who were you the last time you were happy/five or ten years ago/ when you were at school?" is a good follow-up question, as is "Who/what would you like to be?" From the answers to these questions, it is possible to discuss the way forward. What were you good at? What were your aspirations when you were growing up? Did you believe in anything? What inspired you?

That we all have a creative side is often not recognised. During their formative years, for many people, only certain aspects of their personality and interests were encouraged. Activities that bring pleasure or emotional release may be discouraged. Derogatory asides will often colour approbation and celebrations in even the happiest homes. In some households, there may have been little understanding of a child's urge to be creative.

It's always important to keep in mind that you don't have to be "good" at something to be allowed to enjoy it.

She was a maths teacher, and had been promoted to the post of Deputy Head. Her successes in this were always praised and rewarded. By most people's definition of the word, 'Niamh' was a success. She was fiercely private, and when she first came to the group she came across as a very stern, organised lady who had her life under control.

But self-harm had become a problem. She said that she hated the school, she hated the kids, she hated her colleagues and above all, she hated herself. She had become more and more isolated in recent years, and had struggled against suicidal thoughts for a long time. It made her angry when the group facilitator asked the question, "Who or what did you want to be when you were fifteen?"

She had been found to be very good at academic work – especially maths – as a teenager, and this lay behind her anger. But the real answer to the question of what she had wanted to be was "a dancer". There were some smiles in the group at the thought of this middle-aged lady learning to belly dance, but of course, many ladies of all ages do this.

Her parents had actively discouraged any impulse towards creativity when she was young, and it was made clear that this was a lesser occupation. But work and more work wouldn't make her a fully-rounded person. She never did take up belly dancing, but began to experiment with ceramics, and produced marvellous, brightly coloured pots.

After some weeks, working with professionals one-on-one and within the group, Niamh found that she could see enough of her original self to understand that she needed creative activity in her life. She was able to recover fully from her struggle with self harm once she had regained balance in her life and learned to keep a space for the creative.

Moving On

Moving away from the fears, cycles and problems that keep the sufferer emotionally trapped is often the goal of therapy. Recovery must be at the pace that they feel they can move, and always in small, achievable milestones.

The self-harmer won't always respond positively to things like timescales and concrete goals. A good support-person will always be able to remind them that bad days happen. If this can be accompanied by gentleness, kindness and possibly even physical contact, all the better. Even the smallest achievement – which should never be disparaged – can be praised and emphasised, in order to lay the renewed foundations of self-esteem.

This may be frustrating for the would-be carer, but moving on is not about the friends/parents/professionals ego, and we should stay away from the situation if we cannot hold back when necessary. It can do much more harm than good if someone else imposes their idea of recovery on a person struggling with self-harm. A positive cycle of mental health can fortunately be formed quite quickly when the individual begins to move on.

There are bad days, of course. In order to maintain an understanding of the progress they have made, someone who is recovering from self-harm should always be encouraged to keep a diary. There is no linear progression when it comes to recovery. Not every day has to be better than the last – what's important that the ratio of bad days to good moves slowly to favour the good.

Things can only get better. Any form of progress should always be reinforced and celebrated in our journey towards moving on.

A good support-person will always be able to remind them that bad days happen. If this can be accompanied by gentleness, kindness and possibly even physical contact, all the better.

Summing Up

- If we want to help someone we care about to steer away from the road that could well lead to suicide, it is vital that we help the individual return to good mental health.

- Once mental health is restored or improved, we can start to move back towards a complete life and full general health.

- "Becoming the person you were meant to be" is a good goal to keep in mind during recovery.

- There is no shame in struggling.

- What is guaranteed is that as you begin to recover, you will emerge as bigger and stronger than you have ever been in your life, and the demons that haunt you will be vanquished forever.

- Bad things happen in life, and we all respond to them.

- Good mental health can always be approached, especially given patience and support.

- The many factors that contribute to good mental health are available to everyone, however unlikely that may seem, and anyone who struggles with self-harm issues can find one or two small items amongst them.

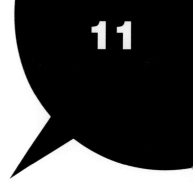

11

Discussing Our Activities

Hopefully you've kept track of the activities and scenarios we explored over the course of this book, because we're going to go through them now! If you skipped any, go back and take a look at them now, before reading this chapter.

There are no right or wrong answers, since we all approach any study from an individual point of view.

Activity One

Give some thought to the reasons you decided to read this book. Write down any specific questions that you would like to be discussed. As you work through the chapters you may find information that surprises or even challenges you. Be sure to leave a space under each so that you can fill in the answers as you come to them.

Write down any reasons you can think of that a person might start self harming.

Take note of anything you come across that surprises you or challenges your preconceptions.

Everyone has their own reasons for wanting to understand more about self harm, so this preparation exercise asked you to examine your own reasons. Before reading any non-fiction book, this is always a good exercise to employ to ensure we get the most out of the text.

Activity Two

Think about the following questions.

- What sort of feeling is produced when you are faced with evidence of self harm?
- When dealing with situations involving self harm, what are the words that you habitually use?
- How do you act or physically respond to these situations?
- Does your facial and body language suggest a sense of scorn or superiority?
- Do you always use positive and acceptable phrases?
- Is this more marked in certain situations or with certain (types of) individuals?

2.1: Practising Empathy

If you believe that others are denigrating your feelings, or even laughing at them, you will find that the situation is much more difficult to cope with.

- Picture a very difficult time you've gone through, when several bad things may have happened very close together. The events themselves may not have been the worst possible things in your life, just consider your feelings. Perhaps the difficulty came from people around you failing to respond or act in a sympathetic manner. You will find that your emotional pain increases if you have a sense of being trapped in a bad situation and cannot see who to trust or turn to.

- Next, think about how you would like people to have responded to you, and what you would have liked to have happened. What would you like them to say to you? What would make you feel less alone at this time? What should the people be saying?

- How would you like to be treated in a situation like this?

These exercises focus on improving our empathy towards people who are going through situations that we haven't ourselves experienced. It is easy to increase the damage to their self-esteem, if we respond with anger and frustration. There are bad times in every life, but for some the opportunity to talk and resolve the issues is not readily available.

The darkest times in life can easily become overwhelming, and we can begin to appreciate this when we attempt this exercise in empathy. Then when we are trying to help someone who self-harms, it is easier to remember what we might most usefully say. When we are struggling, there are certain things that we do and do not want to hear, and we can identify these through this activity.

Activity Three

- Remember a time when you have been the target of a bully. They may have been in your family, at school or in the workplace. To start this exercise, take note of your role in the situation, where it took place and how old you were.

- Consider the person in the role of "bully".

- Who were they to you? What was their role?

- In what way were they bullying you?

- How did the situation pan out?

- Do you feel any anxiety or sadness about the memory?

- If that person was in front of you now, what would you say to them?

- Now that life has moved on, how would you describe your bully's character?

- Did you recognise what they did as bullying at the time?

How would you feel today if you met someone who was cruel to you years ago? While the chance to tell them what you think of them may never present itself in real life, it is still good to imagine what you would say to them, to prove that they no longer can hurt you. This exercise asks you to remember a situation in which you were bullied or mistreated in the past, whether or not you recognised it at the time.

Unresolved situations like these can often result in us carrying unresolved baggage around for years. And even after a number of years, it is still possible to process and deal with these unwanted emotions.

Activity Four

Julie must leave her school, because her family is moving to another part of the country. Now she finds herself afraid of the new situation. She no longer feels that she is loved – or even deserves to be loved, and has started to think that the world would be better without her. Her appetite is affected, and she begins to suffer from vomiting and headaches.

She grew up with a strong group of friends and while she has always been quiet, she was also comfortable and cheerful. Now, she is afraid and nervous around her new classmates. She has no experience of establishing new friendships. Her father only really admits there is any problem, when Julie is found to be cutting herself. She wears long sleeves and hides the evidence.

Her mother doesn't know how to help, but she's worried about the changes she's noticed in her daughter.

Which groups within the new school is Julie at risk from? What might make her realise that they are a negative influence? What help is needed to stop this negative cycle? How is Julie's new environment affecting her body image? How do you think Julie is likely to respond to negative attention in school? How can Julie move to a better social environment and escape her current problems?

In this scenario, our character is forced to leave behind her friends and the situations she is familiar with when she changes school. This becomes a negative spiral, resulting in vomiting, headaches, weight loss and eventually cutting. Julie's body and body image are both affected by antagonism from a group of girls, who cause her a great deal of anxiety.

Although it may be hard to answer, the question "What help is needed to stop this negative cycle?" is a crucial one. Further ideas about how to improve this situation may occur to you as you move through the book, so it may be helpful to return to this activity a number of times.

Activity Five

Give some thought to the idea of a 'meaningful occupation' and how you feel about it. There is no doubt that these include finding a way to describe yourself. It may include voluntary work, or something creative or simply active. The occupation can include anything that gives you a sense of satisfaction and achievement, and does not have to be paid work.

It is important to allow time to reflect on what might work as a 'meaningful occupation' to you. What makes this sort of occupation meaningful are the positives it brings. What positives would your meaningful occupation bring? It might bring the chance of new friends, the ability to say 'I am a swimmer/writer/carpenter/dancer etc.' or something to occupy your brain, and give you a strong sense of self-image.

Think about the benefits that you can expect from your choice. You can begin to pursue this activity as soon as you allow yourself to discover what this would be, by thinking of ways forward.

This activity asks readers to think about the idea of a 'meaningful occupation' and what their own meaningful occupation might be. It is easy not to recognise how key this can be to self-image, and how strong a support it can be to good mental health, unless we do this consciously. Your choice of occupation will determine the benefits that it brings, so it's a good idea to also list these.

In the future, it would be a good idea to make sure your meaningful occupation becomes a consistent part of your life, and to maintain an awareness of the concept as you move forward.

Activity Six

Give some thought to your own early years. Nobody's childhood is perfect, so don't be shocked if it isn't all happy memories! For the purpose of this exercise, make a list of the positives that you took away from your childhood and disregard the negatives.

- Picture a different childhood for yourself. Think about parents who are addicts, alcoholics, or severely depressed. Imagine that you, as a child, become aware that one of your parents is self harming.

- Now decide what you might need to do need to do, to undo the psychological damage that this unhappy experience causes.

- How might this affect your self belief, values, thoughts and attitudes?

This may take some time – give it as much thought as you need.

This activity asks you to imagine an unhealthy, negative childhood, while recalling the positive, healthy aspects of your own upbringing. Later in life, it becomes very difficult to break free of the bad mental habits and beliefs that developed during childhood if you grew up in a bad situation. This exercise aims to help you imagine what these beliefs might include and how persistent they might be.

Again, there are no right or wrong answers, since what works for each of us is a very individual thing.

Activity Seven

For this activity, we'd like you to make two lists. In one list, include everything you can think of that brings you pleasure. In many ways, the more silly the better. Try and remember to include people who help you, and be as detailed as possible.

- The second list should include possible distractions, such as those mentioned above, or some creative ideas of your own.

- Make these lists very neat and easy to read, and display them somewhere you can see them often.

- Think of the person you are most likely to turn to in a crisis, and tell them about these lists. This means that when terrible thoughts overwhelm you, they can remind you about your lists and encourage you to do things that will make you feel better.

This book mentions the idea of 'ways forward' a number of times, and the two lists that you make in this exercise should form the basis of your ways forward.

Activity Eight

Could you direct someone to more information or a self-help group? If someone we know begins to self-harm, what can we do about it? Do you know how to communicate that you are here to listen to that person? How might she respond?

- Make a list of the things that you think it is most important to do.

- Think of phrases that could help here, and create a list.

- Create a third list of the things that you should avoid saying or doing.

If you needed help, how would you like to be treated? Discuss your ideas with someone else.

8.1: In Their Shoes

Take a moment to consider…

- How desperate must someone be to do this to themselves?

- What could happen that might cause you to consider self harm?

- What responses to our situation would cause you more emotional harm?

- In what way might you hurt yourself?

- What responses would you be desperate to hear if you ended up reaching this point?

8.2: For the Professionals

If you are a health professional, try to ask yourself these questions on a regular basis.

- Can I find a calm stillness within myself, which I can call upon so that I act gently and professionally in a difficult situation?

- Can you use this so that everyone (patient, relatives and professional team alike) learn from the experience?

- Is anyone around likely to interfere with my efforts to calm the situation, and if so can they be delegated to deal with some other aspect of the situation?

- What can we all learn from how we operated?

- What do I understand by open questions?

- What does the term 'listening skills' mean to me?

- What is the best way to deal with a situation in a way that will calm the sufferer if I believe I can only spare them a certain amount of time?

- Can I avoid language that suggests prejudice or judgement when I document these discussions? (Keep in mind that the words you include in medical records are considered a legal document.)

- After the discussion, will we have time to debrief and make notes?

- In what way do you use your tone of voice, words and body language? Imagine yourself to be the team leader, and consider what guidance you would give to someone less experienced than yourself to help them.

These exercises are designed to further prepare ourselves to deal with a crisis situation. It is especially important to have an understanding of this if you are a healthcare professional, or a volunteer who deals with individuals in crisis on a regular basis. It is crucial to know how best to respond to others in a time of need. Health professionals should consider the words they might use, and practice these upon a colleague, who will then tell them how that question made them feel.

We should never take it personally if the questions we ask aren't answered. This may simply not be the right time. While questions are a valid way to communicate concern, we are never owed an answer. A better way forward is to offer gentle, calm support by simply being with the individual. It is vital that we are able to adapt to suit the individual's needs, and we should reflect this in our communication styles.

Activity Nine

Give some thought to the people in your caseload (if you are a medical professional). You have the potential for a group if you can identify things that some of your patients have in common. You may already have your group if you are part of a voluntary support network. Before you begin, however there are certain questions to be asked.

- How will you explain the group to potential members, and what might you say to persuade them to join?
- What might follow?
- What are the rules and boundaries?
- How often will you meet? Where?
- What protocols might you want to put in place?
- And what is the optimum number of members, excluding yourself and your co-facilitator?
- Who can you rely upon to co-facilitate with you?
- What does this group hope to achieve?
- Is it something specific or more general?

- Do you and your co-facilitator disagree on any points?
- Will your group be mixed or single-sex?
- Will people be able to join at any point, or will it be a closed programme?
- Will you keep a record of the discussions?

The group will not founder within a few weeks if you are able to answer these questions before you begin, as this means that structure is in place and you are ready to resolve any issues.

Inconsistency will damage trust and can be very destructive, wiping out all progress. The questions in this exercise may seem too simple or obvious to bother with, but in fact a group will fail if it is not clearly thought through, before it has begun. Someone who self-harms is likely to be offered group work as a cornerstone of their treatment. These individuals are often in a very vulnerable state, and need to know that the facilitators are not going to change the rules and boundaries half-way through a programme.

They need facilitators who know what they are doing and won't treat them like guinea pigs.

Ten to twelve members is generally considered to be the best size for a group of this type. Any more would be too difficult to manage and for members to feel ownership of. A good range of personalities and experiences is necessary, and a group with ten to twelve members is most likely to provide this. Members may not be able to get anything out of a group session with too few members, as this can lead to one individual beginning to dominate the group.

If someone begins to dominate in a group with a good number of members, facilitators will be able to regain control of the situation by diverting the conversation to other members in the group.

Activity Ten

The things that Ellie used to enjoy have all lost their appeal recently - she has been lacking in energy for a while, and has lost interest in her friends. Nobody knows that she has started cutting herself. She is beginning to cut deeper and deeper. She was shocked by the pain at first, but feels she is better at handling it now. One day, her family has to call an ambulance when she is found bleeding from a serious cut.

- Who will Ellie have to talk to?
- Will someone listen?

- How open will she be?

- What would be a good, positive thing to draw her attention to, about herself?

- How might her parents react? What are they feeling?

If you have experienced this scenario for yourself, or with someone you care about, you will know what a dreadful experience this can be.

Ellie's trip to Accident and Emergency is the subject of this activity. Health professionals will be aware that there is no time and space allocated for support or counselling in A and E, and it can easily appear that this is a dead-end situation with nothing to offer, except a deepening sense of shame. A good department should be able to refer an individual to the mental health team, and this should be offered.

This is likely to be the character's most vulnerable moment. Finding oneself in A and E should be a wake-up call, to both patient and family. It is possible to take something away from this situation, however, if the right questions are asked. Few departments do not have the Samaritans' number displayed on the wall, and if someone has found themselves in need of medical attention, they do need someone to talk to.

If you or someone you care about ends up in A&E and is not offered a referral to the mental health team, this is something you can request. Local support groups can also be found through The Samaritans if you tell them which area you live in. It is time to resolve this problem, right here and right now.

Activity Eleven

She was a maths teacher, and had been promoted to the post of Deputy Head. Her successes in this were always praised and rewarded. By most people's definition of the word, 'Niamh' was a success. She was fiercely private, and when she first came to the group she came across as a very stern, organised lady who had her life under control.

But self-harm had become a problem. She said that she hated the school, she hated the kids, she hated her colleagues and above all, she hated herself. She had become more and more isolated in recent years, and had struggled against suicidal thoughts for a long time. It made her angry when the group facilitator asked the question, "Who or what did you want to be when you were fifteen?"

She had been found to be very good at academic work – especially maths – as a teenager, and this lay behind her anger. But the real answer to the question of what she had wanted to be was "a dancer". There were some smiles in the group at the thought of this middle-aged lady learning to belly dance, but of course, many ladies of all ages do this.

Her parents had actively discouraged any impulse towards creativity when she was young, and it was made clear that this was a lesser occupation. But work and more work wouldn't make her a fully-rounded person. She never did take up belly dancing, but began to experiment with ceramics, and produced marvellous, brightly coloured pots.

After some weeks, working with professionals one-on-one and within the group, Niamh found that she could see enough of her original self to understand that she needed creative activity in her life. She was able to recover fully from her struggle with self harm once she had regained balance in her life and learned to keep a space for the creative.

Many people appear to succeed in life, but find an inner emptiness which seems never to be filled. Eventually we forget what they were, but our minds and bodies still mourn their loss. You may think Niamh's situation is an uncommon one, but it isn't. We are all creatures of many parts, and this is a lesson we must take away from Niamh's story. Some of the most important parts of our lives can sometimes become neglected, and this is especially true of 'successful' people.

If we allow ourselves to be creative, we can begin to establish ourselves as human beings again. Being human without creativity and all the joys it can bring can be exceedingly difficult. Creative activities can demolish the self-harmer's belief that they are 'less than human'.

Help List

Emergency Helplines

If you are suicidal or experiencing a crisis, you can call these numbers to speak to a counsellor. If you'd rather, you could also travel to your nearest hospital's emergency room and tell a nurse or doctor there what's happening.

Al-Anon UK

www.al-anonuk.org.uk
Address: Al-Anon Family Groups UK & Eire, 57B Suffolk Street, London SE1 0BB.
Tel: 0800 0086 811 (Helpline)
Contact form: www.al-anonuk.org.uk/send-an-email/
Al-Anon Family Groups UK & Eire aim to support anyone whose life has been affected by someone else's drinking. They organise meetings in all major towns and cities in the UK and Ireland, and are committed to being there for you when you need help.

Alateen

www.al-anonuk.org.uk/alateen/
Address and email: Same as Al-Anon.
Tel: 020 7593 2070 (Information line).
Alateen is a group aimed at the teenagers whose lives are affected by someone with a drinking problem. It is organised by Al-Anon.

Alcoholics Anonymous

www.alcoholics-anonymous.org.uk
Address: Alcoholics Anonymous, PO Box 1, 10 Toft Green, York YO1 7ND.
Tel: 01904 644026 (Office hours only); 0800 9177 650 (Helpline).
Email: help@aamail.org
Alcoholics Anonymous is a "Fellowship" whose sole concern is the personal recovery and continued sobriety of individual alcoholics who come to them for help.

APNI – Association for Post-Natal Illness

apni.org

Address: 145 Dawes Road, Fulham, London, SW6 7EB

Tel: 0207 386 0868

Email: info@apni.org

APNI offers support for those suffering from postnatal illnesses such as postnatal depression. They also encourage research and aim to raise public awareness of the illness. You can contact them by telephone or email. The Samaritans or Family Lives (0808 800 2222) can be contacted if you need urgent help outside of office hours.

Broken Rainbow UK

www.brokenrainbow.org.uk

Address: PO Box 68947, London E1W 9JJ.

Tel: 0845 2 60 55 60

Email: Mail@brokenrainbow.org.uk

For LGBT+ victims of domestic abuse.

Bully Free Zone

www.bullyfreezone.co.uk

A website which aims to "raise awareness of alternative ways of resolving conflict and reduce bullying". It is no longer being updated regularly, but has a good list of resources on its "Resources" page.

Childline

http://www.childline.org.uk

Address: NSPCC Weston House, 42 Curtain Road, London EC2A 3NH.

Tel: 0800 1111

Contact form: www.childline.org.uk/registration/

Childline is a free, private and confidential service where children can talk about anything that is bothering them.

Community Mental Health Team

Local service, part of the NHS. Referrals via GP.

Ditch the Label

https://www.ditchthelabel.org

Address: Ovest House, 3rd Floor, 58 West Street, Brighton, England, BN1 2RA.

Tel: (01273) 201129

Contact form: https://www.ditchthelabel.org/contact/

An international bullying charity which provides support, produces research and creates campaigns for change.

Drinkaware

www.drinkaware.co.uk

Address: Drinkaware, Finsbury Circus (Salisbury House), 3rd Floor (Room 519), London EC2M 5QQ.

Tel: 020 7766 9900

Email: Contact@drinkaware.co.uk

Drinkaware is an independent charity working to reduce alcohol misuse and harm in the UK.

Gingerbread

www.gingerbread.org.uk

Address: 520 Highgate Studios, 53-79 Highgate Road, London NW5 1TL.

Tel: 0808 802 0925 (Helpline)

Email: Membership@gingerbread.org.uk

Gingerbread provide information to help single parents support themselves and their family.

MIND

http://www.mind.org.uk

Address: Mind Infoline, PO Box 75225, London E15 9FS.

Tel: 0300 123 3393 (Infoline)

Email: Info@mind.org.uk

MIND provides advice and support to empower anyone experiencing a mental health problem.

Netmums

www.netmums.com

Address: Netmums, Henry Wood House, 2 Riding House Street, London W1W 7FA.

Forum: www.netmums.com/coffeehouse/

Netmums is the UK's most relevant, inclusive and supportive parenting community, welcoming millions of parents every month to their forum, parenting content, recipes, local listings, product reviews, email newsletters and courses.

NSPCC

http://www.nspcc.org.uk

Address: Weston House, 42 Curtain Road, London EX2A 3NH.

Tel: 0808 800 5000 (Helpline)

Email: help@nspcc.org.uk

The NSPCC work across the UK, Channel Islands and Isle of Man to protect children today and prevent abuse from happening tomorrow.

Rape Crisis England & Wales

rapecrisis.org.uk

Address: Suite E4, Josephs Well, Hanover Walk, Leeds LS3 1AB.

Tel: 0808 802 9999 (12 – 2.30pm and 7 – 9.30pm)

Email: rcewinfo@rapecrisis.org.uk

Rape Crisis England & Wales (RCEW) is a feminist organisation that supports the work of Rape Crisis Centres across England and Wales.

Refuge

http://www.refuge.org.uk

Address: 4th Floor, International House, 1 St Katharine's Way, London E1W 1UN.

Tel: 0808 2000 247 (Helpline)

Email: helpline@refuge.org.uk

Refuge supports more than 6,000 clients on any given day, helping them to rebuild their lives and overcome many different forms of violence and abuse; for example domestic abuse, sexual violence, so-called 'honour'-based violence, human trafficking and modern slavery, and female genital mutilation.

Respect

www.respect.uk.net

Address: The Green House, 244-254 Cambridge Heath Road, London E2 9DA.

Tel: 0808 802 4040

Email: abigail.jones@respect.uk.net

Advice and support for perpetrators of domestic violence who want to stop being violent and abusive.

Samaritans

www.samaritans.org

Address: Chris, P.O. Box 9090, Stirling, FK8 2SA.

Tel: 116 123 (Helpline)

Email: jo@samaritans.org

Samaritans is a unique charity dedicated to reducing feelings of isolation and disconnection that can lead to suicide.

Women's Aid

www.womensaid.org.uk

www.thehideout.org.uk (for children)

Address: PO BOX 3245, Bristol BS2 2EH.

Tel: 0808 2000 247 (Helpline)

Email: helpline@womensaid.org.uk

Women's Aid have been at the forefront of shaping and coordinating responses to domestic abuse since 1974. They consist of over 180 organisations, providing almost 300 local lifesaving services to women and children across the UK.

Glossary

Addiction
A physical and mental inability to stop consuming a drug, activity, substance or product, even if it is causing physical or emotional harm.

Adolescent
A young person who is in the process of developing from an adult to a child.

Affect
Medical term for emotions. When affect is said to be flattened, the emotions are not registering normally. Individuals feel cut off from the world and from everyday feelings about it. They feel that their responses are not as they should be.

Body Dysmorphic disorder; (BDD)
A mental disorder characterized by a distorted body image, and also by obsessions about perceived physical shortcomings.

Denial
A mental defense mechanism in which someone refuses to believe a fact that they cannot emotionally cope with. This may be despite overwhelming physical evidence. There are levels of denial, including a tendency to minimise the importance of an event. Denial is sometimes also referred to as abnegation.

Eating disorder
A mental health condition which creates an unhealthy attitude towards food, which can have a major impact on your everyday life as well as affecting your health in the long term.

Endorphins
Tiny protein molecules, produced by the body. These are part of the body's natural challenge to pain, and are produced in times of physical stress.

Generalised Anxiety Disorder; (GAD)
A long-term condition which causes individuals to experience intense anxiety around a wide range of situations and issues, rather than just one event.

Holistic
Concerned with the 'whole' rather than component parts. Holistic care or therapy is based therefore upon the belief that mind, body, social factors and spirit are all interlinked, and that we are not effectively cared for if only one of these aspects is emphasised. This approach is now recognised as the best way of providing support, in any situation.

Homeostasis
Steady state; the balanced parameters that the human body lives within, and the mechanisms to maintain that balance.

Mental health

The combination of someone's emotional and psychological wellbeing.

Obsessive Compulsive Disorder; (OCD)

A mental health condition which features obsessive thoughts and compulsive behaviours. It can develop at any age, and affects people of all genders.

Paralysis

The loss of muscle function in part of the body, resulting in the inability to move that part.

Paranoia

An excessive tendency to suspicion, and (very often) the belief that someone aims to harm us.

Pathologies

Pathology is the study of disease.

Projection

The tendency to attribute distressing emotions about oneself to someone else. (For instance, an unfaithful wife or husband may believe that their spouse is unfaithful.) Projection skews the individual's world-view to a more acceptable set of scenarios.

Psychiatric

Relating to mental illness and its treatment.

PTSD; Post Traumatic Stress Disorder

Caused by extreme stress, which may be physical, emotional or a combination of both. Several features, including hyperarousal and re-experiencing of the trauma (perhaps as flashbacks or nightmares). A numbing or flattening of affect and phobia may also develop.

Self-harm

The act of intentionally causing harm to one's own body, usually as a result of emotional distress.

Syndrome

A collection of signs and symptoms.

Sources

Caponecchia, Wyatt. Preventing Workplace Bullying. Routledge, 2011.

Carter M, Thompson N, Crampton P, et al, 'Workplace bullying in the UK NHS: a questionnaire and interview study on prevalence, impact and barriers to reporting', BMJ Open 2013;3:e002628. doi: 10.1136/bmjopen-2013-002628.

Clark, M. Managing the difficult child. Northcote House, 1999.

Department for Education, 'Behaviour and discipline in schools: Advice for headteachers and school staff', 2016. Download: www.gov.uk/government/publications

Department for Education, 'Bullying in England, April 2013 to March 2018: Analysis on 10 to 15 year olds from the Crime Survey for England & Wales'. 2018. Download: www.gov.uk/government/publications

Ditch the Label, 'Bullying Statistics 2018 & Annual Bullying Survey'. Download: https://www.ditchthelabel.org/research-papers/the-annual-bullying-survey-2018/

Grant, Biley, Walker (editors). Our Encounters with Madness. PCCS Books, 2011.

James, Stephen (June 26–28, 2008). "A Forgotten Right? The Right to Clothing in International Law" (PDF). http://anzsil.anu.edu.au. New Zealand Society of International Law.

Maslow, Abraham (1954). Motivation and Personality. New York: Harper. pp. 236.

Skegg, K. (2005). Self-harm. Lancet 336: 1471

Thomson, J. (2018). The Essential Guide to Bullying. Peterborough: BX PLANS LTD.

United Nations Press Release: Access to Safe Water Fundamental Human Need, Basic Human Right, Says Secretary-General in Message on World Water Day (2001). https://www.un.org/press/en/2001/sgsm7738.doc.htm

need2know